T0184983

# Personal Response Systems: An International Report of a New Home Care Service

# Personal Response Systems: An International Report of a New Home Care Service

Andrew S. Dibner
Editor

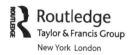

Routledge
Taylor & Francis Group
New York London

*Personal Response Systems: An International Report of a New Home Care Service* has also been published as *Home Health Care Services Quarterly*, Volume 13, Numbers 3/4 1992.

First published 1992 by The Haworth Press, Inc.

Published 2020 by Routledge
605 Third Avenue, New York, NY 10017
2 Park Square, Milton Park, Abingdon, Oxon OX14 4RN

First issued in paperback 2021

*Routledge is an imprint of the Taylor & Francis Group, an informa business*

## Library of Congress Cataloging-in-Publication Data

Personal Response Systems: an international report of a new home care service / Andrew S. Dibner, editor
p. cm.
"Has also been published as Home Health Care Services Quarterly, Volume 13, Numbers 3/4, 1992"-T.p. verso
Includes index
ISBN 1-56024-272-8: (acid-free paper)
1. Personal emergency response systems. I. Dibner, Andrew S. (Andrew Sherman), 1926-.
RA645.75.P47 1992
362.1'9897–dc20                                    92-25580
                                                         CIP

ISBN 13: 978-1-138-97823-2 (pbk)
ISBN 13: 978-1-56024-272-7 (hbk)
ISBN 13: 978-1-315-82538-0 (ebk)

DOI: 10.4324/9781315825380

# Personal Response Systems: An International Report of a New Home Care Service

## CONTENTS

# ABOUT THE EDITOR

**Andrew S. Dibner, PhD,** is considered the Father of Personal Response Systems (PRS) in the United States. He first created the "lifeline" concept in 1972 while on sabbatical at Duke University and has since devoted his career to the development of this service. In 1974, Dr. Dibner and his wife Susan, a sociologist, founded Lifeline Systems, Inc., the leading company in PRS in the world. He has performed numerous studies of the system's effectiveness and has promoted its acceptance by government and health care providers nationally and internationally. Dr. Dibner's background is in clinical psychology and as a professor at Boston University, he specialized in the psychology of aging.

# Foreword

Susan and Andrew Dibner introduced me in the early 1970s to the concept of a personal emergency response system which could assist many frail older adults to continue to live independently. They were post-doctoral research fellows at the Duke University Center for the Study of Aging and Human Development when they conceived and began to develop Lifeline. Lifeline in their view was not just an emergency alarm system; it was a potentially efficient as well as effective way for frail older adults and their caregivers to keep in touch. Keeping in touch in an unobtrusive way, they guessed correctly, would increase the probability that many frail older adults could continue to live with appropriate independence and with a sense of security. The Dibners also understood correctly that the persons who often needed the most reassurance were the caregivers, particularly caring children of the older adult living at a distance.

In developing Lifeline the Dibners were ahead of the times in several ways beyond understanding who it was that needed assurance. When children at a distance contemplate the danger for a frail parent living alone, they understandably consider restricting the freedom of the parent in the interest of safety. The resulting restriction, sometimes leading to institutionalization, is the price frail parents are expected to pay for giving risk-aversive children a sense of security. The Dibners also understood that in the increasingly cost conscious environment of the 1970s and 1980s any proposal for a new service would have to be demonstrably cost-effective. Lifeline from the beginning has been carefully evaluated in terms of its efficiency and effectiveness. Consequently, one can currently say with confidence that personal response systems like Lifeline are surprisingly low cost, are widely perceived as user-friendly, and as part of comprehensive care management programs, tend to reduce care system cost while providing maximum independence for users. That is a winning combination of outcomes for any technology.

This book provides information from a large number of countries that the experience in the United States has been duplicated elsewhere. Personal emergency response systems have a demonstrated capacity to keep frail older adults in touch and to assist in keeping many frail older individuals in the home-like environments they prefer. The accounts of this successful application of technology are particularly appealing because technology in the modern world has sometimes had a very visible darker side. Health

*ix*

care technologies that sustain life can also sustain life relentlessly without dignity, and at very high cost. Technologically sophisticated living environments can become an interpersonally sterile substitute for human caring. There is more and more evidence that, regarding technology in health and human services, more is not necessarily better. The development of efficient, effective personal emergency response systems in a growing number of countries worldwide is evidence of a technology that serves people.

What does the future hold? Personal emergency response systems will surely thrive because they meet personal and societal needs in a cost-effective way. The proportion and number of frail older adults are increasing in all industrial societies and family structures capable of supporting dependent elderly are changing. Changing family structures do not mean that family members care less about older members. It does mean that more women are in the workplace and that the generations are inclined to live separately. It means that geographic mobility and suburbanization of cities ensure that even caregivers in the same community with those for whom they care do not necessarily live next door. New ways of keeping in touch are required.

In caring for older adults, care managers will increasingly make personal emergency response systems an integral component of care plans. This inclusion is already occurring in societies that have national systems of care but remains problematic in societies, such as the United States, that continue a complex mix of public and private service provision and financing. But even in the United States, one observes an increasing number of communities that make service available.

The flexibility which characterizes personal emergency response systems will encourage an increasing number of innovative extensions of a good idea. One already discovers discussions and applications of "smart houses" in which the same system that keeps a frail older adult in touch with sources of care can keep caregivers in touch with indications of environmental temperature, smoke, and the operation of medical devices.

Personal emergency response systems do not solve all or even most of the problems of providing appropriate care for frail but independent older adults. But such systems provide an important dimension of care for a significant minority of frail older adults and their caregivers who want reassurance but also maximum feasible personal freedom.

*George L. Maddox, PhD*
*Chair, Duke University*
*Council on Aging*
*and Human Development*

# Introduction

Andrew S. Dibner, PhD

## THE BEGINNINGS OF PERSONAL RESPONSE SERVICES

With the quickened pace of electronic inventions of the 1960's the technology of personal communications fascinated me. It was at last possible to have reliable, low-powered, inexpensive devices programmed to be simply activated to send messages and to control other devices. The simplest automatic dialers became available for telephone communication. In Sweden, England, and the United States, at almost the same time, inventors applied this new technology to a serious problem–protection of frail and disabled people who lived alone. Using a small, portable radio transmitter in their home, a frail person, in an emergency situation, could activate an automatic call, by telephone or by radio to a neighbor or a help center.

The devices and the service they provided took on many generic names, e.g., medical alert, care phones, community alarms, social alarms, emergency response service (ERS), personal emergency response service (PERS), and personal response service (PRS), The reader will find many names here, but *Personal Response Service* (PRS) will be the most commonly used because the term implies more than emergency or medical uses alone.

Since, in the 1970's, all the developed countries were facing the same, grave demographic changes, viz. a burgeoning of the oldest segments of the population and the concomitant strain on the health care system, there was a ripe atmosphere for experimenting with any means to strengthen the caring resources, and to help threatened people to remain living in their own homes rather than in institutions.

In the socialized countries of Western Europe both the national government and local authorities quickly saw the potential benefits of the new devices and in many locations worked them into their home care systems.

Andrew S. Dibner is affiliated with American Lifeline Institute.

*1*

In the United States, which had the barest and most fragmented of government sponsored home care support, the growth of PRS was instead fueled by the private sector through direct-to-the-consumer sales or rentals, often through the auspices of community hospitals.

All countries have policies aimed at decreasing costly institutional care and increasing home care. Personal response services therefore became an important new home care service rapidly growing in all reporting countries and obviously serving to prolong independent living.

PRS prolongs independent living primarily due to psychological benefits, both in the user and family. It provides a great sense of reassurance, a sense of security that gives users and their family members more confidence when alone, night or day.

World-wide, actual use of PRS today ranges from below 1% to 12% (U.K.) of the elderly population, with several countries reporting 3% (Sweden, Canada, Holland). But estimates of potential use presents a very different picture. Some suggest that 50% of those over 75 may need the service.

For PRS, distribution methods differ depending largely on the social and economic organizations of different countries. In countries with nationalized medical care, governments are involved either at local or regional levels, e.g., housing or social service units provide PRS. In countries where there are government subsidies, often partial payment is due from the user. Screening and referral is most often based on medical criteria. Increasingly, however, subsidies are declining and private pay increasing.

The United States is unique in its use of hospitals to distribute PRS, and funding today has been largely private rather than government sponsored. However, in the United States, there has been increasing inclusion of PRS among Medicaid home and community care services and in supportive services for public housing of the frail elderly.

## AN INTERNATIONAL SYMPOSIUM

As a psychologist and gerontologist with long term interests in the effects of environmental supports on the health and welfare of aged and disabled people, Susan Dibner and I invented the Lifeline PRS system in the United States in 1973, and founded Lifeline Systems, Inc., the largest PRS manufacturer in the United States. In 1986, with L. Dennis Shapiro, Chairman of Lifeline Systems, I founded the American Lifeline Institute as a non-profit organization to pursue research and education about issues involved in aging successfully.

The American Lifeline Institute's first project was to sponsor the *First International Symposium on Emergency Response Services for Frail Persons Living Alone* in Washington, D.C. May 31-June 2, 1990, the fruits of which are the papers in this volume.

Eighteen presenters from 12 countries responded to our call for papers. Each writer was experienced in this young field; they represented greatly varied backgrounds, from university professors to social agency directors to marketing directors of manufacturing concerns.

I offered each presenter a list of topics by means of which they could describe the development and status of PRS in their country. The list included demographic trends, technology, structure of PRS services, economics, operational issues, benefits to consumers and the health system, and expected future developments. Many chose to cite data and examples of their nation's response to the many topics on that list. Their responses are here in this volume.

This volume, therefore may be considered to reveal many snapshots in time showing the status of this new service in nations across the world. The reader will learn, for the countries covered, not only the needs, extent of service provided, financing, etc., but will also, to a great degree, see how the different countries attempt to integrate this new service (sometimes not too successfully) into their health care system. Both PRS and each nation's view of its role in health care and aging emerge as subjects in this volume.

The final chapter peers into the future of this service, both in terms of its technology and its relation to other aspects of health care and other needs and markets. The agreements, disagreements and major issues which arose in the conference come to the foreground here.

## IN APPRECIATION

Without the generous support of many organizations and persons the conference, sponsored by the American Lifeline Institute, could not possibly have taken place. We are deeply grateful for the financial and administrative support of Lifeline Systems, Inc. under the leadership of L. Dennis Shapiro and Arthur Phipps, and the Boards of Directors of both Lifeline Systems and the American Lifeline Institute.

The Symposium received major support from The Charles A. Dana Foundation and significant support from the US National Institute on Aging, the Colonial Penn Insurance Company and the Dibner Fund, for which we are very thankful.

Also of considerable help by co-sponsoring the Symposium were the American Red Cross, National Institute on Aging, National Council on the Aging, American Association of Retired Persons, National Association of State Units on Aging, National Association of Area Agencies on Aging, National Clearinghouse on Technology and Aging, and the United Nations International Institute on Aging.

The American Lifeline Institute would especially like to acknowledge with thanks the spirited, patient and competent work of Ann Marie Yetten, Ted Wayne and Deborah Cutter in making the Symposium successful.

Thanks are also due to the Human Sciences Press, Inc. which anticipated this book by publishing excerpts of the Symposium papers in the 1991 Spring/Summer issue of the *International Journal of Technology and Aging*, Vol. 4, No. 1, and authorized their inclusion in the full length papers that are available here.

# CANADA

# Emergency Response Systems–
# The Canadian Perspective

## Luis Rodriguez

I am pleased to be with you today, because I know we all share a common interest in exploring ways of helping older people, and disabled persons, maintain or restore their independence.

My presentation will focus on three aspects: first, I will talk about the most significant socio-demographic changes taking place in Canada; second, I will tell you about my own findings on the potential of Emergency Response Systems (ERS); and third, I will inform you about the most recent Canadian initiatives relating to emergency response services.

Canada is experiencing unprecedented demographic changes. It is expected that the senior population[1] in general, and the number of people aged 75 and over in particular, will increase significantly over the next 40 years. Today, just over one in ten Canadians is a senior citizen. By the year 2031 nearly one in four Canadians will be 65 or older.

However, we find a more significant change when we look at the number of older seniors who are most likely to need supportive environments. Today 4% of Canadians are 75 years of age or more. By the year 2031, when the baby boom generation[2] moves fully into the seniors ranks, there will be as many people in the 75 plus age group as there are over 65

Luis Rodriguez is affiliated with the Canada Mortgage and Housing Corporation, Canada.

today. If prevailing trends continue over the next 40 years, the 85 plus age group will triple from one-quarter of a million, in 1986, to three-quarters of a million in the year 2031.[3]

A more dramatic picture of the demographic changes in Canada can be seen when we compare the proportion of seniors to the proportion of people between 13 and 19 years of age. In 1971, there were almost twice as many teenagers as there were seniors. Today, there are as many seniors as there are teenagers. If current trends continue, by the year 2031 there will be nearly 3 times as many seniors as teenagers.[4]

Shifts in the dependency ratios will be experienced in the 1990's. The society will be a mature society with a "Baby Boom" generation entering its middle age, and a growing number of families that will more likely be required to provide more care for their elderly parents than for their children, or possible for both.[5] The generation following the baby boomers will certainly have more older people to look after. Consequently, more and more Canadian workers are likely to face the challenge of balancing work and family responsibilities.

We have also been experiencing over the past several decades a significant increase in the participation of women in the labour force.[10] The participation rate of married women in the labour force alone increased from 11.2% in 1951, to 56.9% in 1986.[5] Since women have traditionally been the primary family care-givers, it is reasonable to assume that the substantial increase in their participating in the labour force may have already resulted in a greater number of workers who are looking after their parents or grand-parents. It is also apparent that the increasing involvement of women in the labour force is starting to create a vacuum in many community groups that for many years have relied on women volunteers to provide services to the elderly population.[6]

There are other significant changes taking place in Canada. For example, the fertility rate has been declining since the early 1960's (3.9). It is now (1.7) well below the required rate to maintain a stable population in the long run without large offsetting increases in net immigration.[7]

Declines in fertility, coupled with an increase in the number of lone-parent families, most of which are headed by women,[8] have resulted in a decrease in the average family size in Canada, from 3.9 people in each family in 1961 to 3.1 in 1986.[9]

The economic need for both wife and husband to work in order to meet their family support commitments is on the rise.[5] It is also apparent that geographic mobility among adult children who seek new or better job opportunities is increasing. These trends are likely to reduce the traditional resources for informal support.

The health of Canadians has been improving significantly over the past 50 years, and an increasingly positive attitude towards physical fitness is being reflected in the older age groups.[3] Particularly in recent years, Canadians have been paying more attention to personal habits with regard to smoking, exercising and diet. If these trends continue, older Canadians could remain healthier and more active to a greater age.

There have also been significant gains in life expectancy, both at birth and at the older ages. According to the latest estimates,[11] baby boys and girls born in 1986 can expect to live an average of 73 and 80 years respectively. By 1999, it is estimated that life expectancies of men and women will reach close to 75 and 82 years respectively.[12] Canadians are living longer and this is likely to result in an increased number of adult children with older elderly parents.

According to some American studies, gains in life expectancy have also added to the years during which elderly people experience health problems. Canada can, therefore, expect significant increases in the number of seniors with chronic disabilities.[13] They will have special needs.

One of the fastest-growing groups of Canadians consists of people who live alone. In 1986, 25% of people age 65 and over were living alone (more than three-quarters, 77%, of them were women). If existing trends continue, by the year 2001, 35% of Canadians aged 75 and over ($\pm$1,700,000) will be living alone, up from 30% in 1986.[14] Living alone is the biggest risk factor that forces a frail or disabled elderly person to move into an institution.[13]

In a 1986 national survey,[15] 13 percent of Canadians reported some level of disability. Just over 45 percent of Canada's elderly population said they had some difficulty in carrying out one or more of the Activities of Daily Living (ADL). Most of these older Canadians now live in their own homes (renting or owning); however, the percentage living in private homes, decreases as they age. For example, while 96 percent of all disabled seniors between 65 and 69 years of age live in their own homes, only 57 percent of those over 85 live in private homes. Increasing limitations on their activities is one of the most important reasons why elderly people give up their homes to move into nursing homes or institutions.

Changing attitudes towards many aspects of life is another significant development in our society. Many speakers at a recent international conference held in Canada[16] reported that many frail elderly people and disabled persons would prefer to live independently in their own homes for as long as possible. At a more recent provincial conference,[17] it was noted that seniors want to be self-supportive, and that they want to improve their opportunities for independent living. The many social and economic benefits of enabling elderly and disabled people to remain in their homes were also discussed at these conferences.

The health, social and demographic changes that I have just highlighted will have significant implications in the future. There will be a need to maximize the potential of available traditional resources for informal support; there will be a need to maximize the effectiveness of available resources for formal support; and there will be a need for secure and supportive environments that can enable elderly and disabled people to maintain or restore their independence.

Technology, including Emergency Response Systems (ERS), provides an enormous potential to meet some of the needs.

Studies indicate[18] that most people do not fear "growing old" as much as they fear becoming chronically ill or frail. The ability of older people to remain functionally independent, or to be minimally dependent, can influence their quality of life at home, in the workplace, and within the community.

At Canada Mortgage and Housing Corporation (CMHC), we have been exploring the potential of Emergency Response Systems for enabling seniors and disabled people to maintain their independence at home.

The results of our preliminary work were consolidated in the publication "The Study of the Emergency Response Systems for the Elderly." This publication describes generically the hardware and monitoring services that were available in Canada as of 1988; discusses the potential role of emergency response systems for older Canadians, including a preliminary cost-benefit analysis; and presents the generic criteria that define appropriate technology for older people.

Following this publication, several provincial agencies and private sector organizations have expressed interest in developing and demonstrating ERS which incorporate the features identified as being most desirable.

CMHC also worked with the Province of Ontario on a study of Emergency Response Systems. The work included developing performance specifications for a system that met the requirements of the study steering committee, and evaluating products and systems from 22 manufacturers located across Canada, the USA, and western Europe.

I would now like to take a few minutes to tell you about what I call "my own findings" on the potential of ERS.

The first case is that of a young elderly couple who live in a 2-bedroom apartment, in a seniors' condominium development where the average age of the residents is about 78 years. While viewing their apartment I noticed an ERS device on the wall, and asked how useful it was for them. The man told me that they will never want to live in an institution, and that they wanted to make sure that they could count on assistance if needed.

In a visit to a congregate housing development, I was discussing the "do's" and "do nots" with the administrator. There was a pull-on emergency call system in each apartment which the residents could only activate when in the bedroom or in the bathroom. The administrator noted that one of the residents, who had a bad hip, had once fallen down on the floor in the middle of the living room and had not been able to call for help, even though the system had a two-way communication feature, because the resident was unable to get up and reach the activating device on the wall.

This situation could have been prevented if an appropriate system had been chosen.

The last case is one of an older senior who lives alone in a 3-bedroom single family house. This senior who sometimes uses a wheelchair, or a walking cane, has adapted the house to her own personal physical needs. She recently subscribed to an emergency responsive system, and when I asked her what the system did for her, she responded: "It gives me confidence, and this helps me to stay put."

Many representatives of the industry, ERS program managers, and support and home care providers think that ERS are "a wonderful thing." Recently, I asked the director of an ERS program[19] if she knew what her clients thought of ERS, and she told me this:

- between 10 to 15% think ERS inhibit their freedom. Many refuse them because they do not want to give their house keys to the respondents.
- between 80 to 90% think ERS are liberators, and
- Ninety-five percent of their relatives think ERS are a great idea.

Many people also feel that the availability of effective and affordable ERS could play a major role in enabling frail older people and people with physical and developmental disabilities to live outside an institutional environment. Last month, I discussed this with some ERS program managers and they told me a few case studies, including the following:

In Saskatchewan,[20] an 81 year old man, living alone, with angina, hypertension and arthritis, had 11 admissions to hospital during the last year prior to receiving an ERS unit. The average length of stay was less than 2 days per admission. During the following year, after having received the ERS unit, he was admitted to hospital for the same medical problems only two times. The lengths of stay were similar.

In Ottawa, Ontario,[21] an 82 year old woman, with both of her legs amputated, was determined to remain in her conventional rental apartment. She lived alone. Her only daughter, who lived 400 km away, visited her twice a year. She decided to stay put in her apartment, with the help of an ERS unit and the necessary support services, and lived there for two years until she died.

From my involvement in various study committees, and my discussions with a number of program administrators and ERS users, I have come to the conclusion that "choice" plays an important role in the area of emergency response systems. It is important that a wide range of systems and products be made available to meet a wide range of needs. These choices should include a variety of designs, a variety of technical features, and a variety of costs. Manufacturers could make a substantial contribution to widen the existing range of choices not only by making different products with different features available, but also by making their products compatible with the products of other manufacturers' so that more than one type of product can be accommodated in one single monitoring station.

In my discussions with program operators, I have also learned that electronic emergency response systems are generally very reliable. However, as one program manager[22] pointed out, electronic equipment can always go wrong. For example, what happens when the computer goes down, or when the telephone line does not work? It is important, therefore, that all concerned, including users and their relatives, be aware of the limitations of technology. Legal agreements are usually good tools to ensure that the parties concerned understand what ERS can and cannot do for them.

Research is also indicating the circumstances in which ERS can be useful. In 1988, Dr. Anthea Tinker told Canadians that ERS were very successful in England, but only when provided along with other things as well. In a very recent survey in Canada,[23] it was found that while an ERS in itself would not keep older people in their homes longer, it could along with other support programs, help to do just that.

A recent evaluation study here in the USA among 550 seniors[24] concluded that ERS are a beneficial home care service for elderly persons who are living alone, severely functionally impaired and not socially isolated. This study also found that ERS can reduce costs of health care and improve quality of life.

In Canada the need and demand for ERS appears to be growing tremendously. Today, close to 25,000 people use ERS from a variety of programs and systems that are available across the country. A number of arrangements to obtain services and equipment exist including paying monthly fees for monitoring service and equipment rental, and purchasing equipment and paying monthly fees for monitoring services only.

I would now like to tell you about a number of initiatives that are taking place in Canada:

**In Nova Scotia**, a self-help group of 600 seniors has just completed a survey[23] among 730 seniors (which represents 10% of the total senior population of the study area) who live in a variety of housing forms both in rural and urban areas. The survey was coordinated out of a nursing home,[25] and one of the three surveyors in a 79-year old senior.

The study team felt that "personal security" was one major factor affecting seniors' decisions to stay in their homes, and decided to identify the potential need and demand for electronic and/or social emergency response systems. The study originated on the hypothesis that a successful home care program should include an appropriate emergency response system.

Thirty of the 730 households interviewed said that they needed and wanted an emergency response system. This, in technical terms, means that 4.1% of the total senior population in the study area would need and want an ERS. Ninety seven households said they wanted and were willing to pay for an ERS, which, again, in technical terms means that 13.3% of the total senior population in the study area would want and be willing to pay for an ERS.

Of the seniors who needed and wanted an ERS, 73% lived alone, 47% lived in rural areas, 53% lived in urban areas, 57% lived in their own homes, and 37% lived in seniors' buildings. Seventy-seven per cent felt that they needed an ERS for health reasons, the balance said that they needed it for both health and security reasons. Many seniors expressed a need for an ERS because they were 75 or more years of age, a time of life when "they feel they can expect anything to happen."

Of the seniors who wanted and were willing to pay for an ERS, 60% lived alone, 27% lived in rural areas, 73% lived in urban areas, 71% lived in their own homes, and 23% lived in seniors' buildings. Fifty-seven per cent of the seniors felt they wanted an ERS for health reasons, 26% said they wanted it for combined health and security reasons, and 17% wanted it for security reasons alone.

The study team concluded that an emergency response system should be an important and necessary component of a home care program designed to enable seniors to stay in their homes for as long as possible. Such a program, they feel, could also reduce the number of hospital days currently taken by seniors, and should be implemented as quickly as possible. The study team also concluded that an appropriate ERS should combine both an electronic component and a social component (such as a friendly telephone call a day), and that it is important that such a system be affordable for all seniors and disabled persons.

In Saskatchewan, a study is being undertaken to investigate the feasibility of the city of Regina,[26] in collaboration with its fire department, to offer combined emergency fire and medical alert response services to all citizens of the city, from the child running out to play leaving an appliance turned on, or people at risk in commercial buildings, to an older senior living alone.

All emergency calls would be monitored 24 hours a day by a central response station located at the fire department. When a medical emergency call is received, it will be transferred to the local ambulance dispatcher's office.

One of the advantages of offering emergency response services on a universal basis is the potential for reducing the cost to consumers due to a possible larger number of subscribers. The initial number of subscribers has been estimated at 3,471, including both residential and commercial buildings (179).

Possible subscribers to the Regina initiative include 60 residents of an enriched housing development at **Pioneer Village**,[27] a continuum of care retirement community offering a wide range of accommodation and support services options for seniors. These seniors, whose average age is 81 years, live in self-contained apartments in two 2-storey buildings which are interconnected by a service-rich internal street. Thirty-three of these seniors pay rent in building A, and 27 have purchased a life interest in building B. Many of them have one or more chronic conditions, some have arthritis or diabetes and others have difficulties in undertaking one or more activities of daily living. This integrated approach, which will combine appropriate design, access to community-based support services and emergency response systems, has an enormous potential to enable seniors to remain living independently for as long as possible.

Emergency response systems are also becoming very popular in rural areas and small towns. For example, the **St. Peter's Hospital in Melville**, Saskatchewan, has been operating a program [28] for seniors who live in small communities, since October 1987. Most of the (225) subscribers are older seniors[29] who live alone (70%) but do not want to live in a nursing home. Thirty percent of the subscribers live with their spouses, or somebody else, who in many cases is also frail, or has one or more disabilities.

The cost of the home ERS units is $660, and there is a monthly fee of $20 for monitoring and maintenance services. Usually, community groups, service clubs, or non-profit organizations provide the funds to make ERS units available to seniors. The number of units available, however, is limited and their distribution is based on criteria established by a multidisciplinary assessment team. The assessment team allocates the units on a priority basis to those most in need at the time of application. In all cases ERS services are provided along with the necessary support services.

Following the first six months of operation of this program, a questionnaire was mailed to all subscribers or their families, for an evaluation. Seventy-two per cent of these questionnaires were completed and returned. The results indicated that the following objectives of the program had been met:

- to help ensure that an emergency response will be provided when required and within a reasonable time;
- to reduce anxiety about living alone due to fear of medical and/or environmental emergencies;
- to enable frail elderly and disabled persons to live independently in their homes;
- to facilitate early discharge to the community;
- to reduce unnecessary institutionalization in health facilities; and
- to increase people's willingness to extend themselves and perform normal activities when alone at home.

All respondents indicated that they felt more secure at home with ERS. While most subscribers said that they wore the activating device at all times, a few said they occasionally removed it. There were two real emergencies, and 29 false alarms. Three responses were initiated due to client inactivity.

In Alberta, the provincial government implemented an innovative emergency medical alert program [30] on January 1st of this year. This program is being delivered through the housing division of Alberta Municipal Affairs. The principal objective is to help seniors remain living independently in their homes for as long as possible.

The program provides low and moderate income senior renters[31] with grants of up to $700 to purchase an approved medical alert home unit from an approved medical alert agency. Consumers are responsible for the installation costs and the monitoring services and maintenance fees charged by the agency to which they subscribe. Some agencies charge $25 for installation costs. The average monthly fees for monitoring and maintenance services is $CDN 25, but these fees range between $0-to-32 depending on the level of subsidies that subscribers receive from the agencies. Eighty percent of the agencies charge the average monthly fee for monitoring and maintenance services.

Senior homeowners, or disabled persons, may apply for grant money under one of two other new programs, "Seniors Independent Living Program" or "Home Adaptation Program," and if eligible, some of their grant money under these programs may be used towards the purchase of an approved medical alert unit.

The program also provides one-time grants of up to $CDN 20,000 to help new or existing non-profit agencies establish or expand emergency medical alert networks. Non-profit or commercial agencies wishing to participate as an approved supplier of medical alert equipment and services must meet established program guidelines.

As of the 25th of April of 1990, 700 applications had been approved, and close to 600 Emergency Medical Alert units were in use.

Between 1,500 to 2,000 units were in service under this program by the end of 1990. While it is expected that 1,000 additional units a year will be approved in the initial subsequent years, future demand may stabilize as the needs of the target group are being met.

Most subscribers under this program are older seniors living in the community in private apartments, or in the homes of their children. There are a few who live in seniors' buildings where meals and supervision services are provided. Forty per cent live in rural areas and 60% live in urban centres.

In most cases ERS and other support services complement each other to enable seniors to live independently. Many relatives have encouraged their seniors to get an ERS unit because of the potential benefits for both subscribers and their relatives.

I would now like to tell you about an innovative project being undertaken in Montreal, **"The Shelter Housing Project"**[32]; but before I do that, let me give you some background on the issues that this project is addressing.

Changes in the ability of many seniors to maintain independent lifestyles in rent-geared-to-income housing[33] are having significant implications for the managers of seniors' buildings and portfolio administrators across Canada. Activity limitation, inappropriate physical environments, and in many cases lack of access to community-based services are increasing the risks for many seniors of having to move into an institutional environment.

From recent studies in Canada,[34] as well as from several discussions at a series of seniors' conferences being held across the country,[35] it is becoming apparent that many frail seniors still prefer to remain living independently in their homes for as long as possible, and that this is possible if they have the necessary support. In addition, there is a strong feeling that living independently in rent-geared-to-income housing can be a less costly and more welcome alternative to living in institutions for many seniors. The problem, however, is that much of the existing stock of this type of housing is not designed to address the changing needs of seniors as they become older and more frail. The proportion of older seniors in rent-geared-to-income housing is growing significantly–lending urgency to the need to tackle this issue.

"The Shelter Housing Project" is a pilot demonstration designed to address the particular needs of a group of older seniors living in an eight-storey, 10-year old, rent-geared-to-income building containing 77 self-contained apartments.[36] It is a collaborative effort between l'Office Municipale d'Habitation de Montreal, the Department of Community Services at the Montreal General Hospital, and the local community service centre Notre Dame de Grace-Montreal West.

The principal objective of this 2-year pilot project is to test and demonstrate each of the following strategies, and to find out how the overall intervention can help seniors live independently in their homes while maintaining a high quality of life:

- Strategy One: providing an electronic emergency response system program for a selected group of frail elderly residents who live alone, have functional difficulties in undertaking one or more activities of daily living, have medical problems which can cause a crisis (such as a bad heart, diabetes or sudden dizziness), or feel insecure;
- Strategy Two: making the building physically accessible to all seniors and implementing a home adaptation program for those seniors who have functional difficulties in undertaking one or more activities of daily living;
- Strategy Three: Redefining the traditional role of the housing manager as "more of a supportive manager," to ensure that the needs of seniors are met either by the formal or the informal support networks. The new responsibilities of this manager include playing the role of a prime respondent in the emergency response service program.
- Strategy Four: ensuring that seniors have access to community-based support services; and
- Strategy Five: facilitating a better interaction between seniors living in the building and seniors living in the community, to maximize the

efforts of available resources, and to support self-help among seniors.

This pilot project was implemented in November of 1989. Following an initial assessment of the needs of all seniors involved, electronic emergency response units were installed in 32 apartments, minor home adaptations were made in 13 of these apartments, and a community room was made available in the building to facilitate access to community based services for all seniors involved. The average age of those who received an electronic emergency response unit is 84 years.

The cost of the ERS program is being subsidized by l'Office Municipale d'Habitation de Montreal. The cost of installing a home unit is $25. A $20 monthly fee covers the costs of leasing a home unit, receiving emergency response services and maintenance, and receiving a friendly call once a week.

The costs of home adaptations ranged between $22 and $668. Adaptations included small things such as providing a bathtub transfer-seat, or installing new low shelves in a kitchen.

A preliminary evaluation of this pilot project was made in 1990, indicating the two following results:

- Result One: Between November of 1989 and March of 1990, the housing manager received a total of 16 emergency calls. Out of these, 5 were real emergencies; 5 were false alarms; and 6 were from people who needed some help, but not urgently.
- Result Two: It appears that "the feeling of security among those who received an electronic emergency response unit has really increased."

**In Ottawa, Ontario,** The Elizabeth-Bruyère Health Centre has been operating a very successful emergency response program[37] for the last three years. The number of subscribers to this program has and continues to increase very quickly. For example, the numbers increased from 100, two years ago, to 450 today; and this is expected to increase to 600. While most of the subscribers to this program live in the Ottawa area, there are also many who live in nearby towns, and some (10%) who live in rural areas. Most of the referrals for ERS come from the office of the Home Care Program.

The majority of the subscribers to this program (75%) are frail women aged between 80 and 85 years, but there are also disabled people in their early 20's (10-15%), and older seniors in their mid 90's. The age range of adult subscribers varies between 40 and 97 years.

About twenty percent of the subscribers live in single family homes with relatives, seventy percent live in seniors' housing and residential care homes, and close to 5% live in emergency housing for families, and in homes for emotionally disabled children. In the latter case, care attendants are the ones who wear the activating device.

The Elizabeth-Bruyère Health Centre purchases emergency response home units from a supplier at an average unit price of $750, and leases them to subscribers.

Twenty-five percent of the subscribers use two-way-voice units, and seventy-five percent use basic units. Monitoring services are provided from a Central Monitoring Station located at the centre. The Ontario Ministry of Community and Social Services funds 70% of the program's operating costs, excluding purchase of equipment and depreciation. Subscribers pay a $25 fee for installation of the home unit; and a $35 monthly fee to cover the costs of leasing and maintaining the home unit, and receiving the emergency response services. Usually, community groups, service clubs, or non-profit organizations provide funds to make ERS services available to subscribers. Some 23 volunteers help in installing home units, testing equipment, making friendly calls every month to subscribers, and filing and processing correspondence.

During the three years of operation of this program, there have been a total of 4,367 false alarms, and a total of 531 real emergencies (as of the end of April 1990). This indicates that just under 11% of the total number of calls have been real emergencies. Feedback received from the manager of this program indicates that ERS help many people maintain their independence, when provided along with the necessary support services.

**In New Westminster, British Columbia,** the Queen's Park Hospital offers a community based non-profit program[38] designed to enable a number of people to remain living independently and safely in their homes. Subscribers to the program include individuals with health problems, elderly people, disabled persons, those recently discharged from the hospital and those who live alone.

The program serves a catchment area where 20% of the population is already 65 years of age or older.

As of the end of April of 1990, the program had 137 subscribers whose age ranged between 52 and 101 years. Close to ninety percent were women, mostly widows, who lived in apartment complexes and seniors' residences. The other ten percent were men. About 40% of these men lived with their spouses or family members.

The Central Monitoring Station at Queen's Park Hospital receives about 65 calls per month. Forty-five of these calls are usually accidental, 11 are non-emergency calls, 4 are inactivity calls, and 5 are real emergencies. About 60% of the emergency calls are caused by falls; the rest are usually caused by a medical emergency, such as a heart attack. The ERS program has made it possible to bring people to the hospital within ten minutes following an emergency call.

Queen's Park Hospital purchases basic units and two-way voice units from a supplier at an average price of $750, and leases them to subscribers. Subscribers pay a monthly fee of $23 for the basic unit, and $30 for the two-way voice units. These fees cover the costs of overhead, and equipment rental and maintenance.

**In Alberta,** the High River Hospital and Nursing Home has been operating a successful ERS program [39] since April of 1983. This program currently serves 45 elderly people and disabled persons who live independently in their homes.

Most of these people are older seniors who live absolutely alone (80%), are afraid of falling, have had a heart attack or stroke, are partially paralyzed or are in wheelchairs. Fifty percent are women and 50% are men. The majority (90%) live in single family houses, some (5%) live in private rental apartments, and a few live in seniors' housing.

Through day-to-day observation and experience, the managers of this program have found that ERS provide many benefits including: (A) reducing anxiety, and increasing confidence, among both subscribers and their relatives; (B) reducing the number of visits by subscribers to the doctor; (C) relieving the need for adult children to send their parents to a nursing home; and (D) saving many lives through timely and appropriate emergency responses.

The Central Monitoring Station is located at the High River Hospital. The hospital purchases ERS home units from suppliers at a price ranging between $450 and $750. Subscribers pay $20 for initial installation costs, and a monthly fee of $15 to cover the costs of renting the home units and receiving maintenance and monitoring services.

**Across Canada,** the interest in ERS by government agencies and non-profit community-based organizations is growing, and several new initiatives are emerging. For example, in the Regional Municipality of York, in Ontario, a committee representing the local hospital, housing operators, elderly and disabled consumers, and the Seniors Citizen's Division of the Regional Municipality, have been working together for the last year to design, develop and implement an ERS program[40] for the entire region.

The Regional Municipality of York, which is playing the lead role on the committee, is looking for a commercial partner to deliver this program. This partner would be responsible for establishing a local monitoring station, supplying the necessary equipment and staffing, installing home units, and making available emergency response services and ongoing maintenance services. The municipality would make referrals through its networks, provide coordination and follow up services, and in cooperation with the Ontario Ministry of Community and Social Services, would provide funds to eligible subscribers to cover the costs of installing the home units, purchasing or renting the home units, and receiving emergency response services and maintenance services.

The Municipality is currently reviewing a number of proposals from several companies, and it expects to be able to implement the program sometime in August of this year. It is expected that close to 200 ERS units would be in operation in the first year. The total uptake for the first 5 years is expected to be 2,000 units.

Costs for services and equipment under this program are very preliminary at the moment. However, it is estimated that those wishing to purchase a home unit would pay a one-time sum of $800 for it, and those wishing to lease a home unit would pay a monthly fee of between $23 and $24. Emergency response services would be available for both buyers and renters at a monthly fee of $20.

The **Canadian Automated Building Association** in collaboration with several other organizations is undertaking a "Study on Applications of Building Automation for Elderly and Disabled Persons." This study will identify opportunities for Canadian firms to participate in the development and marketing of new technologies which respond to the needs of disabled and elderly persons and potentially could be adapted to the building market at large. The objectives include: (A) to assess the nature and size of the potential market in terms of the needs of the current and future elderly and disabled population that could benefit from automated buildings technologies; (B) to identify appropriate conceptual and technological responses to the needs of elderly and disabled people; and (C) to identify the social and economic benefits and costs of building automation for elderly and disabled persons.

Integrated approaches to building automation including emergency response system functions have potential for further helping many seniors and disabled persons live independently in their homes. These approaches, with greater facilities for passive activation, could enable them to undertake the activities of daily living and to monitor many other functions in their homes with increased safety, comfort, security and convenience.

To summarize, significant socio-demographic changes have occurred in Canada over the last 35 years. These changes have implications for Canadians in the future. If current trends continue, there will be an increased need to maximize the effectiveness of available resources in order to address the needs for formal and informal support of older seniors and disabled persons.

From the information presented in this paper, it is apparent that most older seniors and disabled persons prefer to remain living independently in their homes for as long as possible, instead of moving into institutional environments. This is possible if they have the necessary support. It is also apparent that Emergency Response Systems (ERS) are playing, and will continue to play, an important role in enabling many seniors and disabled persons to maintain their independence.

Across Canada, the interest in effective and affordable ERS is growing rapidly, and a variety of innovative initiatives are emerging. Most of these initiatives combine the reassurance of emergency response systems with appropriate physical environments and accessibility to the necessary community based support services. The objective is to help older seniors and disabled persons remain living independently in their homes for as long as possible.

## NOTES

1. Arbitrarily for this presentation, the senior population is defined as all persons aged 65 and over. People aged 75 years and over are defined as older seniors.

2. Those born between 1946 and 1966, from "the Seniors Boom" by Statistics Canada, October, 1986.

3. "The Seniors Boom," by Statistics, Canada, October 1986.

4. Canadian population projections by Statistics Canada.

5. Workers with Family Responsibilities in a Changing Society: Who Cares, by the Canada Employment and Immigration Advisory Council, June 1987.

6. From the article, "Social Agencies Hit by Volunteer Shortage," The Ottawa Citizen, 19 May 1990.

7. Statistics Canada Lecture Series. Can We Afford an Aging Society?, June 1989, by Ivan P. Fellegi, Chief Statistician of Canada.

8. Canadian Social Trends by Statistics Canada, Winter 1987. Women Parenting Alone.

9. Canadian Social Trends by Statistics Canada, Spring, 1989. Changes in Living Arrangements, 1986 Census Highlights.

10. Canadian Social Trends by Statistics Canada, Winter, 1987. Women in Male-dominated Professions.

11. Demography Division, Statistics Canada.

12. The Corporate Response to Workers with Family Responsibilities by the Conference Board of Canada Report 43-89, 1989.

13. Conference Proceedings. Options: Housing for Older Canadians, Halifax, Nova Scotia, October 17-20, 1988. Canada Mortgage and Housing Corporation, "Implications of a Diverse and Changing Population."

14. Canadian Social Trends by Statistics Canada, Autumn 1988, Living Arrangements of Canada's "Older Elderly Population."
15. The Health and Activity Limitation Survey, Statistics Canada, 1986-87.
16. "Options: Housing for Older Canadians," conference held in Halifax, Canada, October 1988, Canada Mortgage and Housing Corporation.
17. "Housing for Saskatchewan Elderly," a Seniors Housing Conference held in Regina, May 1990, Canada Mortgage and Housing Corporation and Saskatchewan Housing Corporation.
18. "Technology and Aging in America." Congress of the United States, Office of Technology Assessment, October 1984.
19. Evelyn MacNamara, Elizabeth-Bruyère Health Centre, Ottawa, Ontario.
20. A case study from an evaluation of the St. Peter's Hospital Program, Melville, Saskatchewan, October 1987 to April 1988.
21. A case study by Evelyn MacNamara, Elizabeth-Bruyère Health Centre, Ottawa, Ontario.
22. Shirley Mann, Director of Volunteer Services/Manager ERS Program, High River Hospital and Nursing Home, High River, Alberta.
23. Report on Electronic Emergency Response Systems, Pictou Council of Senior Citizens and Valley View Villa, Nova Scotia, January 4, 1990.
24. A study of the Effects of an Emergency Alarm and Response System for the Aged, February 1980, Sylvia Sherwood, and John Morris, Department of Social Gerontological Research, Hebrew Rehabilitation Center for Aged, Boston, Massachusetts.
25. The Valley View Nursing Home, Pictou, Nova Scotia.
26. Arvind Bubber, Director of Revenue and Fiscal Services, Regina, Saskatchewan.
27. Ron Reavley, Regina Pioneer Village, Saskatchewan.
28. Brian Kines, Executive Director and Administrator, St. Peter's Hospital, Melville, Saskatchewan.
29. Average age 85 years.
30. Betty Wilson, Coordinator, Agency and Equipment Approval, Senior's Emergency Medical Alert Program, Alberta Municipal Affairs, Government of Alberta.
31. Those people 65 years of age or older, or widows/widowers 55 years of age or older, who live in rental accommodation in Alberta for at least 9 months of the year, and who receive Alberta Assured Income Plan benefits or have a household income of $CDN 25,000 or less for the previous calendar year.
32. Danielle Maltais and Francine Trickey, Department of Community Services, Montreal General Hospital, Montreal.
33. Includes both nonprofit and public housing.
34. (a) Housing and the Health of the Elderly, Metropolitan Toronto District Health Council, March 1988; (b) Habitat-A National Seniors Housing Consultation by One Voice, the Canadian Seniors Network, Ottawa, 1989.
35. Provincial and territorial seniors' conferences being held across Canada between April and September of 1990, cosponsored by Canada Mortgage and

Housing Corporation and the respective provincial and territorial housing agencies.

36. Commonly known as the Monkland Residence.

37. Evelyn MacNamara, Program Manager, Elizabeth-Bruyère Health Centre, Ottawa, Ontario.

38. Kathie Taylor, ERS Program Manager, Pacific Health Care Society, Queen's Park Hospital, New Westminster, B.C.

39. Shirley Mann, Director of Volunteer Services/Manager ERS Program, High River Hospital and Nursing Home, High River, Alberta.

40. Glen Davies, Director, Senior Citizens' Division, Regional Municipality of York, Ontario.

# Product Design
# and Social Implications
# in a Personal Response Program

## Mary Lynne Hobbs

### INTRODUCTION

I would like to begin by saying that, from a Canadian perspective, this symposium is a most important and timely gathering on the issue of emergency response systems. At a time when the seniors population is rapidly growing and independent living is being encouraged, when numerous new ERS products are coming on the horizon, and various governments within Canada are attempting to decide on their role in improving access to these systems, I am both pleased and honoured to share the fruits of our research with you and to benefit from the wealth of information you have to share.

I will be speaking on the approach we are taking and the concerns we have with respect to the technology and service delivery of emergency response systems in Ontario, Canada.

### CHANGING DEMOGRAPHICS

As Luis Rodriguez previously described to you, Canada is a very young country; a constitution establishing it as a confederate nation within the Commonwealth was struck only in 1867.

Ontario is one of 10 provinces in Canada (we also have 2 northern territories). The population of Ontario is about 10 million.

We have close to 1 million people age 65 and older living outside of institutions in Ontario, about 10 percent of the total population. Approximately 4% of the population is 75 years or older. Over 250,000 seniors (or

---

Mary Lynne Hobbs is affiliated with Ontario Ministry of Housing, Canada.

23

25%) live alone. Furthermore, almost half (48%) of the total million seniors report having some type of disability. As is widely true among industrialized countries, the proportion of the population age 65 or older is growing; in Ontario, the proportion is expected to double to 20% by the year 2021.

Among non-seniors, about 16% (700,000) of the adult population in Ontario report having a disability, and 60% of these people have multiple disabilities.

## CURRENT FUNDING SITUATION
## FOR SUPPORTIVE LIVING

Ontario's nursing homes and homes for the aged are funded by the Province's health and social service ministries. As with most governments in recent times, however, Ontario's current direction is to assist seniors to age in place and to live as independently as possible with home and personal support services.

The Ontario Ministry of Housing has a mandate to fund self-contained housing for people who are able to live independently. There are about 43,000 units in seniors' public housing and another 46,000 units in seniors' non-profit projects funded by the Ontario Ministry of Housing. Most assisted housing for seniors today is in buildings dedicated to people age 60 or older, this being the preferred choice of over 90% of seniors. More recently, however, our Ministry has been encouraging the development of housing for those who prefer an age-mixed environment, meanwhile continuing to support seniors-only buildings.

## NEED AND DEMAND

Close to half of the existing seniors' housing stock was built 15 to 25 years ago for the healthy and independent senior. However, instead of moving on to care facilities later in life, as expected, seniors have tended to age in place. Now we find that there are many seniors with health problems and functional limitations living in our buildings.

A study done by the Ministry (Denton & Davis, 1986) in 5 selected housing projects indicated that between 70% and 90% of the tenants surveyed required some assistance with activities of daily living. In one municipality, a survey was done of selected seniors' buildings which found that 80% of tenants felt that an emergency response system would be important or very important to them.

How to ensure that senior citizen tenants can remain independent for as long as possible, while preventing our buildings from becoming institutionalized, is a major challenge facing our Ministry today.

In the broader community, it is estimated that 440,000, or 47% of seniors may be in need of an ERS (i.e., have a disability/age 75 and live alone), and 40% of these may require subsidies (i.e., presently receive only old age security). Another estimated 70,000, or 10% of the non-senior disabled population may be living alone and in need of an ERS, and 32% may require subsidies (i.e., presently receive welfare assistance).

However, experience in Ontario to date concurs with some programs in Europe and the United States that only 3% of all seniors in communities that offer ERS actually use these systems.

### ERS IN ONTARIO: ENTER THE GOVERNMENT

What is the status of emergency response systems in Ontario right now, and what role does the government play in providing these systems? Generally, the private market has been the primary agent to-date in providing emergency response systems, and the user normally pays the full cost. They are not found on drug store shelves, however. Normally, a consumer would contact a distributor or service recommended through a health practitioner, relative or friend.

As Luis Rodriguez has pointed out, ERS is very new in Canada. For years, there have been only a few domestic ERS manufacturers, supplying basic, institutional nurse-call systems or direct digital dialer systems. In the past 2 to 3 years, companies have been proliferating–local firms, and international firms with local branches, subsidiaries or distributors. It is quite exciting to see the range and quality of technology advance so quickly to meet the need for independent living supports.

I often get asked, if the private sector is doing the job, why must the government get involved? We are looking at some type of public involvement primarily because of concerns over AFFORDABILITY, AVAILABILITY, ACCESS ADEQUACY and CHOICE. ERS development has been patchy to date in Ontario:

- ERS services are available only in certain communities to date (and many companies, typically foreign firms, supply equipment without the monitoring services)–the product is of little use without the service!

- where ERS services are available, product empires or monopolies seem to have developed
- products vary considerably in terms of quality, and there are no standards yet established specific to ERS, other than standards set by the Federal Department of Communications (#CS-03) for electronics equipment.
- many seniors find the cost unaffordable–equipment from private firms can range from $400-$1,100 in Canadian dollars; private market monitoring services are generally provided for $15-30 per month excluding equipment rental; with equipment rental, monthly fees range from $20-35.
- lack of consumer information and access to products and services is such that the average senior, doctor or home care worker would have no idea how to access an ERS, what choice is there, and what to look for in an ERS

The Ontario Ministry of Community and Social Services has provided funding for 9 local ERS monitoring services, serving an estimated 500 clients as of October, 1989. Most operate from various homes for the aged. The Ontario Ministry of Health is funding at least 32 such services across Ontario, normally based in hospitals or nursing homes, and serving approximately 5,000 clients. A rough estimate of 3,000 people are served through the private market. Some municipalities have independently chosen to subsidize emergency response systems for disabled persons on welfare assistance in their communities. These costs are shared by the Provincial Government. This is considered a special item, and no standards seem to apply as to which emergency response systems would qualify. In a few communities, service clubs (that is, volunteer clubs that do community work), have undertaken fundraising to help subsidize needy individuals who require emergency response systems.

Clearly, in the absence of a concerted government policy on emergency response systems, Provincial and municipal governments and local communities have responded to the need for ERS on an *ad hoc* basis. Why the hesitation of governments to intervene in this market? Primarily for the following reasons:

- tremendous potential costs, at the same time as we face fiscal restraints
- possibility that less expensive, lower-technology alternatives (for example, postal alert or daily telephone checks) are sufficient for many people

- lack of better data on the long range financial and social costs and benefits (e.g., delayed entry to residential care facilities for the elderly)

## A CLOSER LOOK AT SYSTEMS AND TECHNOLOGY

The Ontario Ministry of Housing in 1987 initiated an ERS Committee (chaired by myself), which was joined by the Canadian Government (represented by Luis Rodriguez), various Provincial ministries, and the Municipality of Metropolitan Toronto. This committee attempted to establish a framework for the study of emergency response systems.

With the assistance of a rehabilitation engineer, Dr. Geoff Fernie, and an electronics engineer, Jack Nissan, the Committee developed Performance Specifications for what we considered an "ideal system."

These specifications reflected our philosophical view that

- *ERS is only one of the supports necessary* to enable supportive independent living for seniors and disabled persons.
- *ERS is very much a human system*, and must respond to the needs of individuals (i.e., must have two-way voice communication which would not only verify an emergency but would reassure the person at home that help is coming).
- *ERS should not be viewed as a medical device* for "frail and sickly people at risk," but rather as an independent living system for anyone desiring reassurance and security; thus, to avoid stigmatization and lend dignity to the individual, we emphasize the importance of aesthetics. The device should be simple, as small and lightweight as possible, attractive, unobtrusive, blend into the home like a common household fixture, and display minimal labeling (none at all, if possible, through the use of different coloured and shaped buttons or perhaps universal symbols).

Even though all evidence suggests that portable devices generally are not worn by users, we believe that a device aesthetically appealing, discrete, light and waterproof may be more popular than believed. One study in Alberta (Woods, 1989) showed that 28% of ERS users living independently in the community liked the pendant least about ERS and 32% did not wear their pendants at all times. The portable device should be available in a variety of styles (e.g., pendant, wristband, pocketclip). We hope to come across a portable device that is or could be built into a person's jewelry.

- *A fixed device should be available for every room or exterior space* (e.g., porch, balcony) within easy reach of a person standing or lying on the floor; a pull cord is thought undesirable because of its institutional connotations.
- *ERS must be useable or readily adaptable for persons with various disabilities* (manual, visual, auditory or mental impairments).
- *ERS should not generally be used in place of a telephone,* for reasons that:

    – over 98% of Canadians have a telephone (although this varies by community);
    – ERS equipment and services are relatively expensive; and
    – ERS operators need to be free to answer genuine emergencies

Nevertheless, many isolated seniors and others use ERS primarily to make human contact. *It is essential to ensure that other community systems are in place to meet the emotional needs of isolated individuals,* such as local friendly visiting programs, and ERS operators should be able to link a socially isolated individual to a more appropriate service.

- *Seniors should have a choice over whom they wish to have contacted in an emergency; the system should be able to program at least 4 telephone numbers, one of which would be a central monitoring station.* Although most people would agree that individuals "at risk" should be guided towards a "top down" approach (i.e., a system that would first alert the central station, which would then contact other personal or emergency resources), we are interested in exploring the potential for a system which has the flexibility to be either "top down" or "bottom up," at the choice of the ERS user. We are curious as to the effectiveness of a system which would observe the following triage format. If responder number 1 picks up the phone, he or she would hear a coded message that would be recognized as a call for help, and may even identify the caller. If responder number 1 is willing to attend to the call, he or she would press digit 9 on the telephone dialling pad confirming this, and two-way voice communication would be opened between the caller and the responder. If the ERS receives no such acknowledgement, it would proceed to dial responder number 2, and so on. It would be crucial to have the central monitoring station as one party on the list of responders, however, in case none of the other responders was available. We are interested in discovering whether this "bottom up" feature would be desirable, as an option for some people, because:

- it is expected to be more popular among rural dwellers, persons of different ethnic backgrounds, and others who rely strongly on their friends and neighbours and who have a great mistrust of more remote, formal services
- It may be the preferred option among seniors and disabled persons who are essentially healthy and Independent and who have a strong support network, but who simply desire a little reassurance and personal contact
- given the high false alarm rates (typical rates are 90-97%), this option would minimize unnecessary reliance on a costly service and leave operators free to attend to genuine emergencies

- *ERS should include a "passive" option*, for example, a non-motion detector, for reasons that:

- many seniors simply refuse to wear a portable device, and thus, the risk remains of an unattended emergency
- seniors have said they fear the possibility of being left for periods of time injured and incapacitated, and
- equally importantly, should they die, they would want the dignity of being found within a short period of time

Some property managers believe that their healthier, more independent senior citizen tenants would find that a requirement to call in to the monitoring station or press a button daily would be intrusive in their lives. This would involve modifying their lifestyle and would give some a feeling of being supervised. The Alberta study suggests otherwise (92% of ERS users in the community felt their ERS was not an invasion of their privacy). However, it is difficult to say how many people reject an ERS for reasons of intrusiveness. Privacy and independence is a strong part of the Canadian culture, especially among the older generation, and emergency response systems would still be viewed by many with mistrust. Such daily requirements would also result in innumerable false alarms when people would forget to call in. One of the greatest technological challenges is to develop a sound "passive" strategy which would pick up all genuine emergencies without causing high false alarm rates.

The matter of high false alarm rates is not altogether straightforward. By "false alarm," I refer to those 90% or more calls which may be considered inappropriate uses of the system, e.g.:

- passive alarm activated when the person is not at home or not in an emergency

- accidental triggering (e.g., person accidentally pressing the button while getting dressed)
- visitors (e.g., grandchildren) playing with the system
- use for social contact which should be satisfied in other ways

Some non-emergency uses of an ERS, however, may be quite legitimate, e.g.:

- person experimenting with their system to increase their confidence or comfort level
- person testing their system for functional reliability

The Ontario Government has put a good deal of thought into what it feels is needed in an ERS, and has sought information from ERS firms at home and abroad as to the systems that are available. It has also looked into existing literature on need and demand. Furthermore, it has been examining the legal and ethical implications of employing various client technologies, including emergency response systems.


### NEXT STEPS

What will we do with this information? At the moment, we are exploring what role emergency response systems play in the context of the wide range of human services and technologies that assist seniors and disabled persons to remain living independently in the community. We are trying to decide on what role the various governments should play in assisting people to obtain access to emergency response systems and services, and under what conditions. To decide on this, we require more information, perhaps from a field study, which would improve our understanding of the cost-effectiveness of an ERS program relative to lower-technology alternatives, the need and demand for such a program, and the requirements for a potential ERS Program in Ontario.

We believe that emergency response systems have tremendous potential in terms of assisting people to obtain prompt help in an emergency and reducing the concern and anxiety of ERS users and their families over living alone.

However, before investing many millions of public dollars in an ERS Program, we need better information on . . .

- In what situations would an electronic ERS be the most appropriate option for an individual? What other program options (e.g., daily check-up calls) would be more appropriate in order to enhance personal security?

• Would ERS on the whole:

– foster a better relationship between ERS users and their families and friends by providing peace of mind? OR
– deteriorate the relationship between ERS users and their families and friends who are part of the ERS responder network by increasing the demands placed on them? OR
– result In increased social isolation because family and friends feel less responsibility? (Results from a CMHC study (1988) of 23 ERS users in Ontario suggest that social contact does not decrease after acquiring an ERS).

• Would an ERS create overdependence on technology where other services would be more appropriate (e.g., medical check-ups, home care, hospitals, care facilities), perhaps creating in the ERS user a false sense of security?
• Would a person's misuse of an ERS immunize responders to a genuine emergency, thereby placing them at greater risk?
• Would ERS delay seniors' entry into nursing homes or homes for the aged?

The CMHC study found that 2 out of 23 ERS users returned home from a nursing home having acquired an ERS, and 30% reported that they would seek other accommodation if they did not have their system. However, one cannot conclude that cost savings would result in residential care, because the supply of care beds falls far short of demand, and most facilities have long waiting lists. Furthermore, one monitoring service operating from a home for the aged in Toronto discovered that very few seniors on its waiting list were interested in an ERS. It was thought that these people required high levels of care and were convinced that their chances of being placed in the home would decrease if they accepted an ERS.

• Would ERS:

– **reduce** demand for emergency services (e.g., hospital emergency department, ambulance, police) and other support services (e.g., attendant care, home nursing care), resulting in rationalized service delivery and more appropriate allocation of scarce community resources? OR
– **increase** demand for emergency and other support services, resulting in greater agency case loads and expanded funding?

- Would ERS reduce the burden on local housing staff in responding to incidents and tenants' personal crises?
- What should be the minimal and the optimal requirements of emergency response systems, should the government introduce an ERS Program?
- Are there circumstances where the "bottom up" approach (i.e., dialling first to family or friends) is more appropriate and desirable than the "top down" approach (i.e., dialling first to the central monitoring station)?
- Would local monitoring stations be more sensitive to ERS users and more cost-effective than regional or provincial monitoring stations?
- What would be the most effective "passive strategy" to ensure that: (a) all genuine incidents are responded to? and (b) false alarms are minimized?

Many questions remain. The Provincial Government is working together with the Federal and local governments to answer some of these questions and decide what involvement we should have in assisting seniors and disabled persons to obtain access to emergency response systems and other human or technological personal security systems. Whatever program we choose would need to address our concerns of availability, affordability, access, adequacy and choice.

In conclusion, the Government of Ontario has made great progress in the area of investigating emergency response systems. But before plunging into a program, we need to answer some fundamental questions. At the risk of studying this issue to death (and Canadians are known to be cautious–or is it prudent?), our investigations will continue.

## REFERENCES

Canada Mortgage and Housing Corporation (1988). *The Study of Emergency Response Systems for the Elderly*, Toronto, Canada.

Denton, M.A. and Davis, C.K. (1986). *Patterns of Support: The Use of Support Services Among Senior Citizen Public Housing Tenants in Ontario*. Ontario Ministry of Housing, Toronto.

Woods, G. (1989). *A Feasibility Study of Introducing Emergency Response Systems to Senior Citizen Lodges*. Edmonton: Alberta Municipal Affairs.

# DENMARK

# Services for the Danish Elderly: The Role of Technical Aids

## Henrik Friediger

How society sees the elderly, and what provision society makes for them varies from country to country. The way we think and act in Denmark is special for us and originates from a 100 year old political and social culture. A culture which has developed in accordance with the Danish landscape and the social movements which have arisen and which still influence the society. In particular a strong cooperative movement among farmers and a strong trade union movement among workers. About 100% of the Danish labour force is organized in unions.

Before I go into details about ERS in the care of the elderly, I would like to outline some main principles and tendencies in the care of the elderly which are dominant right now.

### HISTORY

The development of services for the elderly has been parallel to *industrial* development in Denmark. This can be seen in some of the solutions

Henrik Friediger is affiliated with National Board of Social Welfare, Denmark.

*33*

earlier applied to cater to the needs of the elderly. Principles applied in the industrial sector, such as standardization and centralization were reflected for a long time in solutions in the form of *institutions*. These principles could best be applied by keeping the old people in nursing homes and as far as possible standardizing the services.

But highly standardized care can lead to making the service and care impersonal and not suited to the needs of the individual.

In recent years Denmark has by and large left the standardized institutional solutions. There has been a change of attitude so that the main goal in Danish services for the old and people with a handicap is to reinforce the influence of the individual on his or her own life.

## NEW PRINCIPLES IN CARE FOR THE ELDERLY

These days we start from the needs of the elderly and their ability to decide themselves what service they want. The key-words in Danish services for the elderly today are continuity, self-determination and use of the individual's own resources.

By *continuity* we mean that as far as possible we should be avoided disrupting the lives of the elderly. By *self-determination* we mean that the old people themselves should decide how they want to shape their existence, and by *use of the individual's own resources* we mean that the elderly should use the forces and resources they have. This is important in order to avoid unnecessary passivity in their lives.

"We want to act ourselves–not to be treated."–"We want to handle our own lives."–"General living problems should not be considered as an illness."–These are expressions of some active old people. And these attitudes correspond to the official attitude in the area.

To reach the goals set up, a broad spectrum of provision for the elderly has been established. These options are intended to help ensure that the elderly can remain in their own home even if they have a great need of care. They should also help ensure that the elderly can decide for themselves how they want to be cared for. We are moving *from total care to self-care*.

## FROM NURSING HOME TO OWN HOME

Danish legislation has been changed in accordance with these goals. The relevant bills were passed by the Danish Parliament in summer 1987.

This means that in the future no more nursing homes will be built in Denmark. Instead there will be housing for the elderly, that is, housing adapted to suit elderly people and people with a handicap.

As a general rule housing for the elderly will be built as independent apartments with kitchen and bath and without institutional features.

Emergency response services are installed so that help may be called with short notice in case of sickness, accidents or the like. The residents must feel secure–even in the apartments for the elderly.

The individual apartment must be designed with particular regard to accessibility so that the residents may remain living there even if they get frail and demand more care.

To achieve good results we try to consider the conditions characteristic for the area where the apartment is situated. Both needs and solutions may vary from one community to the other. The new legislation on housing gives good opportunities for integrating housing for the elderly in already existing buildings. In this way it is possible to avoid ghettos.

Since, in the future, services for the elderly will be provided, as a rule, outside institutions, it is important to have provision for the need of the elderly for support. Therefore a broad and varied network of services is essential.

## HELP IN THE HOME

Practical assistance in the home will often be necessary. A round-the-clock service should be available to secure personal assistance and care in the daytime, in the evening and at night.

In Denmark many municipalities have now introduced evening service or round-the-clock service. Connection to such services may be an important condition for many elderly to remain in their own homes. The service has different forms in different parts of the country, but normally they consist in a combination of an alarm unit where help can be summoned, and an arrangement where assistance can be given after previous agreement.

Home help is part of the arrangement. The elderly can be helped with personal care, daily household jobs, and assistance with participation in activities. Furthermore home nursing can be given, free of charge. Home help is also free of charge in Denmark.

## INTEGRATED SYSTEMS AND CULTURE

The development in Denmark tends to form integrated service systems in the municipalities. The home nursing and the home help work together in one system and are combined with provision of physiotherapy, occupational therapy, together with meals-on-wheels.

Unfortunately, I have only time to mention that this whole system is only part of all at the old peoples' disposal. A fundamental principle is that old age is not a disease. That is why we must not only focus on the things you cannot cope with but also look at the resources we all have—even if you are old and fragile. That is why we have to also provide inspiration by means of adult education and other leisure activities.

## THE GOAL IS SELF-DETERMINATION

Our goal is to provide services which guarantee the elderly self-determination and their right to live on their own premises. Here clients need to be involved in the decisions to be taken. When public assistance is needed, we must consider the situation of the individual citizen, and the assistance should be based on confidence and respect for the person in need of assistance.

It is important not to put anybody under tutelage, misunderstanding the need of care. The person in need of assistance should therefore actively take part in the process and realize that they also can depend on their own resources.

Life-long self-determination is a basic principle in Danish policy for the elderly. The goal is to provide a variety of services suited to the needs and desires of the individual. That is so in all fields: health, social services, and a satisfactory cultural life.

## USE OF THE EMERGENCY RESPONSE SERVICE

I will now tell you more specifically about the use of emergency response systems in connection with the very short outline I have given of the Danish model for elderly care.

The housing for the elderly which is to be built in the future instead of nursing homes must provide the means to call help at any time of day or night.

It is also easy for old people living in their own original homes to have an ERS installed. All that is necessary is electricity and a telephone point, which as good as all Danes have in their house or flat.

About 5 million people live in Denmark. About 800,000 or 15% are more than 65 years old.

We have no statistics about the number of ERS in use in Denmark. We estimate 20,000. The increase per year is about 1,500-2,000.

To give the above some meaning, I can tell you that about 47,000 households have permanent home nursing and 135,000 households permanent home helps.

## ACTIVE AND PASSIVE SYSTEMS

You can divide the ERS into two different types: Active and passive.

The user himself activates the alarm of an *active system*, e.g., by pushing one of the pushbuttons installed in the dwelling. Or the resident can activate a portable radio transmitter. Active systems are the most widely used and experience shows that systems of this type are easy to understand and operate.

A *passive system* can be separately installed but may also be a supplement to an active system. The principle of the passive system is that the alarm is activated when a daily routine is not performed within a certain period of time. Examples of this can be opening the refrigerator, flushing the toilet, turning the radio/TV on or off and crossing the doormat.

In practice only the active system is used. Users think the passive system both controls and puts them under tutelage. I have not succeeded in finding one example of use of the passive system for this talk. The ERS demands that users themselves press the button when they need help.

## THREE MODELS

I will now describe 3 models of emergency response systems. They differ not so much concerning instruments but in what happens when the user presses the button. It is of vital importance who the receiver of the call signal is, and the arrangements they set to work.

1. A nationwide emergency service called "Falck," owned by a large insurance company, has developed a concept which they offer to municipalities.

   The concept is that the alarm the users operate is received by an emergency response centre, manned round the clock. The emergency response centre will send an ambulance to the user's address. The ambulance is manned by two people who are trained ambulance-drivers and have had instruction in "first aid," but apart from this they cannot give the user any help. If needed, the user will go to hospital.

The system is safe and effective but very often it will be an overreaction to turn out an ambulance compared with the reason for the user pressing the button. The system is thus rather expensive.

2. Twenty-seven flats for the elderly have been built in a small municipality in Zealand named Suså, in accordance with the new act "Housing for the Elderly." There is a central building in connection to the flats with cafeteria, occupational therapy, physiotherapy, and activity workshops. It also houses the centre for service to the elderly for the entire municipality.

All the 27 flats have an ERS installed and the residents wear a necklace transmitter, a pendant.

There is an unmanned switchboard in the central building, which registers all calls from the residents. From here the calls are switched to 4 home helps and a nurse who are on duty during the day; or one home help and a nurse during the night.

These helpers carry portable receivers which pick up the calls. The display shows who is calling, and the helper goes as quickly as possible to the resident who has called. When the helper comes to the flat they press the button of the fixed transmitter in the flat and the call is registered as answered.

It is not possible for transmitter and receiver to communicate but a tone in the flat indicates that the alarm has been activated when the user presses the button.

Statistics show that the help will come within 5 minutes and not later than 10 minutes after the call was given.

Most residents in the flats for the elderly come from 2 nursing homes which have been closed down. They are in great need of care and service. After an "acclimatisation" period most people are pleased with the new surroundings and the service given.

3. A somewhat bigger municipality in the north-eastern part of Jutland, Sejlflod, has 9,000 inhabitants. About 300 of the elderly in the municipality use a home help and about 100 use home nursing.

It is the policy of the municipality to link home nursing and the use of ERS. Among the 100 users of home nursing 70 have an ERS installed.

The system functions over a closed radio network and the home nurse on duty answers it.

The system allows communication between the transmitter and receiver, and when the old person calls it is a well known voice which answers the call and asks what they can do to help.

The system is very reliable. If the home nurse does not answer after the third signal, it goes on to another nurse, and if no answer is given to a third nurse. If there is still no answer, it goes to a town hall in a municipality nearby.

There is no emergency response centre apart from this safety back up.

It is thought that a lot of money is saved by not having a manned response centre. If a response centre is going to be manned round the clock, it will need a staff of 5. Wages have to be paid before there is money to pay the staff who actually help the elderly.

The system in Sejlflod is not called an emergency response system but only a "call system." The idea is to demystify the use of the system; it is important that the user makes use of it whenever they want to do so.

## COSTS

Now a little about what it costs. A central unit costs about 7,500 dollars, and the unit in the users' flats about 1,200 dollars.

If you choose a solution such as the one in the municipality of Sejlflod, there are practically no running costs.

If you choose the Falck-solution the price per unit is a little less. But the subscription to the emergency response centre costs 100 dollars per unit per year, plus what it costs to send an ambulance, when called for.

## WHO PAYS?

There has been no private market for ERS in Denmark until now. It has been a service provided and paid for by the municipality. But in February this year, Falck launched a new idea where they offer ERS to private people at a price of 60 dollars per month.

## THE FUTURE

There is a great optimism among professional people when you talk about the future. The goal of the Danish policy for the elderly is: Remain in your own home and use your own resources for as long as possible. This means that it will be necessary to develop a technology which will provide people with appropriate help whenever needed. There is great potential for the development of ERS-technology. The only limits on the development of call technology are the imagination. The elderly of the future–like me–are more used to technology than the elderly of today.

Science fiction futures are often shown to us where all are watched through the use of technology. But I think it is reassuring that the old people in Denmark have refused to use the passive system. *They* will decide for *themselves* when the button is going to be pressed. Self-determination for the individual. The future looks promising.

# General and Specific Aspects
# of Emergency Response Systems
# in Denmark

George W. Leeson

## INTRODUCTION

In this paper we shall consider first of all technology developments in general referring where relevant to their impact upon the lives of elderly people. This is followed by a discussion of elderly technology as we see it and anticipate its development from a Danish viewpoint.

In the second section of the paper, the development of the technology of surveillance equipment for elderly persons since the 1970's is considered. The implemented systems and the economic aspects are also discussed.

In the third section of the paper the demographic development in Denmark is considered along with the consequences of this development for specialized housing and technological surveillance for elderly people.

Finally, the changing profile of the elderly population in Denmark in the future is considered based on the results of the on-going "Future Study" carried out by the DaneAge Foundation.

## INFORMATION SOCIETY–POLICIES AND THE ELDERLY

Modern society is constantly undergoing change–a change which is never predictable. The changes that take place today take place faster than ever before and affect the lives of more people than ever before. As far as technology and technological aims in the home are concerned, the intricacies of their development is reserved for the initiated.

---

George W. Leeson is affiliated with DaneAge Foundation, Denmark.

Most recently, information technology and biotechnology have been in the focus of public attention. There is a feeling of the brave new world which entails both unforeseen possibilities and apprehensions.

Social planning at all levels has almost always been plagued by an inherent inability to forecast technological development and as the science of these technologies becomes more and more elitist attempts to forecast development will become increasingly difficult. There is no doubt a danger that technology will create an additional class division of the population: those that understand and control and those that cannot and do not. It is claimed in defence that technological developments will increase production which in turn will increase everyone's welfare and wellbeing, regardless of whether or not they are employed.

Much of the hitherto technological development in various sectors has lead to centralization and rationalization. In many countries, especially the public sector has experienced this centralization. In Denmark this tendency has been particularly strong. The romance of small village schools, of small town hospitals, of happy elderly people surrounded by caring friends and neighbours is quite unable to compete with the efficacy of technology's centralization. Even so, it cannot be denied that technological development has also lead to decentralization bringing improved conditions to more sparsely populated regions.

Technology brings with it new horizons, new challenges. There is a very definite fear that it can remove the personal touch associated with something as simple as the local bank or library which can now be contacted via a home-based terminal. But having said that, this could certainly be an enormous benefit to the large number of elderly people confined to their homes and previously unable to take advantage of such offers. And the prospects of the communicating computer (one with verbal input and output) will ensure that everyone–including apprehensive elderly people– is able to operate these home-based terminals.

As a matter of policy it is imperative then that the elderly are encouraged by courses and other initiatives to be active in the on-going technological development, otherwise they will most certainly risk increased isolation.

The encroachment of technology in our own homes is in fact now widely accepted. Washing machines with built-in computer programmes, microwave ovens, programmable vacuum cleaners and TV-sets and videos etc., etc. Of course, many of these products have made our daily lives a lot easier. There is more time to relax when we are not at work. And even more recently, innovations that have previously been reserved for industry and business have encroached: Alarm systems, speaking clocks, TV-data, personal computers, electronic surveillance. The home is becoming increasingly like the work place.

Home-based activities will undoubtedly benefit many people and perhaps especially elderly persons, but they will also undoubtedly give rise to increased demands for personal social contact.

Before technology arrives and becomes (perhaps) an implicit part of our lives it is imperative to determine people's needs and thereafter find a niche for technology. Of course, we may then risk that the full scope of technology is not exploited right away but it will ensure acceptance and application.

The Danish government has for a number of years now had a policy aimed at ensuring that an elderly person can remain in his/her own independent dwelling for as long as possible. If this policy is to be a success–especially as far as the elderly people are concerned–all the necessary support services that could be needed have to be on-hand to meet the challenge presented by this policy. Support services cover a wide range of things: from home help to district nursing, to provision of meals and to emergency response systems. Especially emergency response systems linked directly to nursing services must be operational and available 24 hours a day. An emergency response system without the needed back-up of services (of all kinds) is a hollow promise of security.

As early as 1982, one of the large Danish provincial municipalities (Næstved) introduced a 24-hour emergency home service for elderly persons in their own homes. This service has since been monitored and evaluated by the local Government Research Institute in Denmark. The first such 24-hour service began, however, in Viborg in 1978 and many other local governments have since followed suit.

Home-based emergency response systems for the elderly benefit enormously from technological developments. In the following section, the development of emergency response systems as we know them today in Denmark is discussed in more detail.

Early systems were one-way alarm systems requiring a physically active involvement on the part of the elderly. All existing systems are naturally extensions of the traditional ones with varying degrees of additional sophistication. Almost all, however, require some form of physical involvement on the part of the elderly person. A simple fall may prevent them from reaching the response system, be it a telephone, a button, a cord, an infra-red ray or whatever.

In effect, the latest technological developments now allow total surveillance of an elderly person in his or her home, thereby removing the need for direct participation of the elderly at all. With this possibility arising, there is a very important issue to be tackled relating to the right to surveillance, the right to register. These problems have to be solved and have to be accepted by all parts, and if this is not the case 24-hour response systems for the elderly based on the best technology may well be out of the question.

## DEVELOPMENT OF EMERGENCY RESPONSE SYSTEMS IN SERVICE FOR ELDERLY PERSONS IN DENMARK

Development in two-way emergency response systems for elderly persons in Denmark can be traced back to the early 1970's. The first developments concerned topics relating to housing and care, philosophy, technology, security and care systems. In this section, we shall look at these developments and give examples of the systems in Denmark as well as some of the economic aspects where relevant.

From the late 1960's to the mid 1970's, Denmark–like most western countries–experienced an unprecedented economic boom which provided a basis for increasing security for elderly persons–especially those very frail elderly persons–with far better housing and care facilities than ever experienced before. Up until that time, elderly persons had managed in their own homes with help from families and only a very small minority who were totally incapable of taking care of themselves in their own homes were admitted to old peoples homes.

Towards the end of the 1960's, modern residential nursing homes began to appear. These were equipped with all kinds of modern technology and aids enabling a very high level of service for elderly people in need of extensive care. At about the same time, sheltered housing was developed for those elderly whose service needs were of a more restrictive nature. However, at that time, there was very little development in the area of provision of service and care for elderly persons living in their own private homes.

In the following years, a third alternative type of specialized housing–different from residential nursing homes and sheltered housing–was developed. This is the so-called congregate housing and is in principle an ordinary dwelling usually in close proximity to a service centre and adapted so that even very physically handicapped persons are able to cope in such a dwelling.

This particular type of specialized housing became extremely popular with both elderly people and local governments when the 1976 Social Assistance Act made it possible to provide extensive services for elderly people remaining in their own homes or in specialized non-institutional housing. This type of housing is publically subsidized and *it is a prerequisite that such housing is equipped with emergency response systems.*

By the early 1980's, it had become the official policy of the Danish government that elderly persons should be able to remain in their own homes for as long as possible. Such a policy requires not only *suitable housing* and a *choice of housing* but also the provision of service and care when needed as well as some systems such as emergency response systems which guarantee a feeling of security.

At the beginning of 1989, new legislation was introduced relating to specialized housing for elderly persons. This new legislation means essentially that no more residential nursing homes will be built in Denmark. Emphasis is now placed entirely on individual independing dwellings in proximity to service centres. The type of environment provided is one with individual dwellings, activities when required and–perhaps more important–service and security at hand.

Since the mid 1980's, the number of residential nursing home places has been falling steadily and this can be expected to continue to do so as more and more of this type of housing is converted to individual specialized housing units for elderly people.

So much for the provision of specialized housing in Denmark–an important aspect in the Danish context as far as emergency response systems are concerned. It should perhaps be mentioned already here that the provision of emergency systems is almost entirely a local government concern as is the provision of the necessary back-up service. Only very recently has there been any sign of private initiatives in this area–not surprising in such a well-developed welfare state.

As far as the development of aid-technology in Denmark for elderly people is concerned since 1970, the early period was characterized as one with traditional one-way alarm systems of the type commonly encountered in hospitals and which became standard in the new residential nursing homes being built at the time.

In 1975, the EGV-Organization together with Falck (a large private Danish Security Company) introduced a two-way communication system designed to ensure that elderly people could remain in their own home with a high level of security and safety than had previously been possible. The system was based on the public telephone system and alarms strategically placed around the dwelling. At the same time as this active system was introduced a passive system was also being developed based on passive activation of alarms designed to coincide with the elderly person's daily routine. Alarms would be set off for example if an elderly person did not activate the signal after a specified length of time. The alarm would be followed up by a telephone-call and eventual help from Falck. The provision of such systems/service was administered by local authorities.

By the early 1980's, these really rather primitive systems were being replaced by much more advanced ones with infra-red rays in cross fields, photo cells, etc., etc., while at the same time the two-way call system had been developed almost to perfection. Advanced telephone systems with cordless radio transmitters and automatic calls to private persons also became more widespread, but still almost exclusively under local authority administration.

The latest developments look towards increasing the operational radius of the response systems. Satellite transmissions of an emergency call to the nearest response centre will near precise location of the person in distress requiring little active involvement of the person. Other systems are activated automatically if the person in question remains in a horizontal position (after a fall) for more than some specified length of time. The equipment required is also rather sophisticated–nothing more than a "watch."

With this technology at hand, elderly persons will in almost all situations be able to alert emergency services. Such an emergency response system would still have to be backed up by a fleet of mobile care units–perhaps installed with personal computer systems enabling them to obtain information about the elderly person in need of help on the way to help them.

As already mentioned, in theory, technological development now allow total surveillance on elderly persons in his or her own home. In fact, the elderly persons themselves need not at all be directly involved in calling an emergency service. However, this does mean that there is an issue to be tackled relating to the right to surveillance and the right to register. These issues have to be solved and accepted by all parts if 24-hours services for the elderly based on the best technology are to be realized.

As far as the systems in use have been concerned, they have probably developed more slowly than technology as such. In the early 1970's, emergency response systems in institutions were very much in line with hospital systems–services within easy reach of the elderly person. And it was only in rare cases that calls were transferred to alarm systems monitored by off-site emergency services. The early emergency response system could only operate within a very small radius.

The development of two-way communication systems made it possible to link emergency response systems to professionally manned emergency centres where the nursing staff could contact the elderly person, establish in advance what the need was and respond accordingly.

The policy of helping elderly people to remain in their own homes as long as possible meant that it was necessary to develop a mobile care and emergency service. Under this system, elderly persons are equipped with an emergency two-way response system linked to a 24-hour emergency service centre either at the local authority service centre and nursing home or the emergency services. These centres are in continuous contact with mobile care centres and thus allow for 24-hour home care.

It should again be stressed, however, that all of the developments mentioned here in Denmark have taken place within the auspices of local authorities. They are provisions of the welfare state. Emergency response systems for elderly persons living in their own private homes and not screened for such a system by the local authority are only now beginning to appear on the market in Denmark as the wishes and the needs of the elderly people begin to change and as the welfare state finds it increasingly difficult to meet the demands of the growing and changing elderly population.

Let us now look at two examples of emergency response systems and their use in practice in Denmark. The first example is one of an emergency response system with the emergency centre based in the district nursing home service centre with sheltered and congregate housing in the area under this centre. This specialized housing comprises blocks of 6-12 housing units purpose-built for elderly or handicapped people scattered around the municipality. Each house is linked to the 24-hour professionally staffed emergency centre at the nursing home with an operational radius of approximately 25 kilometres. This was the very first system of its kind in Denmark and it has now been expanded to cover over 200 housing units. At the time of the study, 86 houses were permanently attached to the two-way emergency response system by the telephone net and 100 houses were covered with pre-coded telephones. Furthermore, there were 45 intermittently coupled mobile 2-way emergency call systems based on radio transmission. The use of the system is illustrated in Table 1.

Clearly the calls have predominantly resulted in a home-help visit (57%) indicating that most of the problems occurring could be solved "quite easily." As much as 20% of all calls were of a purely social nature–needing someone to talk to–something not to be scoffed at. Only 8% of the calls were "critical" in as much as they required more expert help or hospital admission.

The second example is of a 24-hour mobile care service for elderly persons living at home "in the community." This has been evaluated not only in economic terms but also with regard to the efficiency of the system. In short, the research showed not only that the establishment of the

Table 1. Use of emergency response systems

| Results of calls | Wrong calls | Conver- sation | Visit of home help | Calling in of: Nurse | Doctor | Hospita- lization | Total |
|---|---|---|---|---|---|---|---|
| Period | | | | | | | |
| 1st 6 month period | 145 | 194 | 470 | 43 | 13 | 8 | 873 |
| 2nd 6 month period | 118 | 198 | 627 | 51 | 28 | 5 | 1027 |
| 3rd 6 month period | 131 | 165 | 471 | 50 | 21 | 4 | 842 |

24-hour care service was economically viable but that the service was widely approved by the elderly people receiving it. Especially the very old were extremely happy, and approximately 25% of those aged 80 and over made use of the 24-hour care service. It is interesting to note that only 25% of the clients received 50% of the visits. In other words, relatively few elderly persons took a large part of the resources of the 24-hour home care service. There was an overwhelming majority of the elderly people attached to the service who felt that they would not have been able to have managed without this service if they had been dependent on help from family, neighbours or friends. It was also clear too that those involved in the project preferred to remain in their own homes rather than move to a residential nursing home or specialized housing for elderly persons. People attached to the emergency response 24-hour home care service aged 65 and over could be grouped into the following "problems groups":

- Motoric diseases 33%
- Cardial- and circulatory diseases 30%
- Frailty due to old age 25%
- Diseases of the internal organs 15%
- Respirative diseases 11%
- Neurological diseases 8%
- Psychiatric diseases 6%

- Cancer 4%
- Metabolic disorders 4%

At the time of the study in the early 1980's, annual expenditure on home care for elderly persons on the 24-hour scheme amounted to approximately 110.500 Dan.Crs. (17.000 U.S.$) per capita. In comparison, the annual expenditure for someone in a residential nursing home amounted to approx. 225.000 Dan.Crs. (34.600 U.S.$) dependent on the extent of care provided. Furthermore, the cost of long term hospitalization was 940 Dan.Crs. (145 U.S.$) per day.

In the five year study period, approximately 120 persons per year were admitted to residential nursing homes in the municipality. The experience from the 24-hour service would indicate that this number of admissions will decline to 50-60. It was also estimated that the annual number of hospital beds being used by this group of persons will decline by 3000 as a result of the service. In other words, this 24-hour emergency response service for people in their own homes would appear to be saving approximately 5 million Dan.Crs. per annum, but more important it is providing better service and care for elderly people in their own homes.

## THE FUTURE ELDERLY IN DENMARK

Since 1986, the DaneAge Foundation in Denmark has been carrying out a "Future Study" designed to elucidate the profile of the future generations of elderly–persons 40-64 years of age today. The study is primarily based on a national interview study among 1200 people in the age groups. This study and other research projects carried out in connection with the future study have provided a very detailed profile of that part of the population which will constitute the elderly over 60 years of age in the year 2010.

Since the turn of the century, the Danish population has aged considerably from 250.000 people aged 60 and over comprising 10% of the population to over 1 million comprising 20%. In Table 2, the development in the age distribution of the Danish population 1989-2011 is presented. This forecast is one which was made in connection with the Daneage Foundation's on-going Future Study and incorporates the recent developments in mortality, especially for middle-aged and elderly men and elderly women in Denmark.

From the late 1950's to the early 1980's mortality of elderly women decreased very significantly in Denmark–by as much as up to 35% for some age groups over 60.

Table 2. The Danish Elderly Population, 1989 - 2011. Thousands.

|            | 1989   | 2001   | 2011   |
|------------|--------|--------|--------|
| **Males:** |        |        |        |
| 60 - 69    | 232    | 235    | 332    |
| 70 - 79    | 157    | 161    | 177    |
| 80 +       | 60     | 83     | 98     |
| **Females:** |      |        |        |
| 60 - 69    | 262    | 251    | 335    |
| 70 - 79    | 213    | 215    | 217    |
| 80 +       | 123    | 171    | 207    |
| Total population | 5129,8 | 5227,6 | 5292,4 |

Source: DaneAge Foundation, Future Study.

The forecast presented in Table 2 in the case of elderly women is based on a continuation of the development observed since 1960 to the year 2011. For males, the forecast incorporates the effects of improved treatment of heart disease as well as the prophylactic effect of improved diets, more motion, etc.

The results of the forecast show that the number of elderly in Denmark aged 60 and over could well increase from just over 1.000.000 today to almost 1.400.000 in the year 2011–an increase of over 30%. Especially the number of very old people over the age of 80 is expected to increase substantially. The mortality development incorporated in the forecasts result in life expectancies for both men and women of approximately 84 years compared with 72 for males and 78 for females today.

Social policies with regard to care and service for elderly people are faced with something of a paradox. Even though elderly people are great users of public and social service most of the care provided to elderly people comes not from public services but from the family and the social network. This is reflected in the fact that less than 5% of all persons aged over 60 are living in residential nursing homes or specialized housing for elderly persons (see Table 3) so in fact 95% of all elderly persons over 60 years of age are living in their own homes receiving for the most part a minimum of help from public services.

Population forecasts such as those illustrated in Table 2 have lead to a hue and cry and Doomsday prophesies–prophesies that fundamentally

Table 3. Elderly in residential nursing homes and specialized
housing for elderly, 1989 - 2010

Forecast

|                          | 1989   | 2000   | 2010   |
|--------------------------|--------|--------|--------|
| Residential nursing home units | 43.700 | 56.400 | 69.000 |
| Specialized housing      | 10.600 | 37.300 | 70.600 |

Source: Central Bureau of Statistics & DaneAge Foundation, Future
Study

ignore the simple fact that the majority of the elderly population are able to look after themselves. That the number of elderly people can be expected to increase substantially in the course of the next 20 years and that the number of the very old people can be expected to increase significantly and the fact that this in itself will mean an increasing number of elderly people in need of help need not in itself be alarming. The fear is based more on the fact that the public sector is becoming less and less able to meet the increasing demand from the increasing numbers.

What will be the increasing demand for specialized care and services including emergency response systems? It must be remembered that in Denmark, the provision of care and services and especially emergency response systems is for the time being at least a matter for the public services. Elderly persons in residential nursing homes or specialized housing for elderly persons and elderly persons receiving help in their own homes (home help, nursing and emergency response systems) are all under the auspices of the local authorities. There is to all intents and purposes no private enterprise in this area. So when considering the future development in the need for specialized services and emergency response systems, one illustrative point of departure is to look at the expected development in the number of elderly people living in residential nursing homes (taking into account the improved health situation and the declining mortality among elderly people) and the development in the need for specialized housing. Emergency response systems will always be in place in these housing units.

In 1989, as can be seen from Table 3, just under 44.000 elderly persons over the age of 60 were living in residential nursing homes and there were 10.600 units of specialized housing for elderly people. Taking into account the improved health situation of elderly persons and the declining mortality among middle-aged and elderly persons in Denmark, the number of elderly in residential nursing homes can be expected to increase to just over 56.000 at the turn of the century and 69.000 in the year 2010. Furthermore, by the year 2000 it can be expected that approximately 26.000 extra specialized housing units will be needed compared with the figure of 10.600 units today and further to the year 2010 an extra 33.000 compared with the year 2000. Thus, in total, by the year 2010 compared with today, there will be an extra 25.300 elderly persons in residential nursing homes and 60.000 extra specialized housing units for elderly persons. In total, an extra 85.300 specialized units all requiring a high level of housing and service including the latest technological developments. These figures are obviously a great challenge to society–something which most certainly has to be planned already today.


## THE FUTURE
## AND "THE REST OF THE ELDERLY POPULATION"

In the preceding section, we looked at the development in the elderly population and especially at the development in the need for specialized housing and–as the situation stands today–specialized emergency response systems as well as other forms of care and service. Even when restricted to this quite limited proportion of the elderly population requiring such specialized care and service there is a vast increase. There are certainly signs in the welfare state in Denmark that the state will not be able to continue to meet all needs and that therefore an increasing amount of private initiative will be experienced. This is already true in the field of the emergency response systems where private emergency services and insurance companies are beginning to offer such systems to elderly persons living in their own homes and not receiving such systems from public services.

Is this something that can be expected to continue and is this something that the future elderly population will require?

Part of the Future Study carried out by the DaneAge Foundation has also looked at the future elderly and their profile and their attitudes towards service and technology.

It is quite clear that the elderly of the future will be totally different and will make different demands from the elderly population of today. Although all these demands will be very different they need not necessarily be more expensive for society. Certainly, the future elderly will be more active, healthier, live longer, be better educated, economically better off, have better housing conditions, be more independent, be used to determining their own lives and making their own decisions. They are also much more politically active and used to organizing themselves in political pressure groups. During their younger years when they were establishing families and pursuing their careers the welfare state was riding on the crest of the wave. All the things we now materially take for granted appeared on the scene during those formative years for the future elderly. They are not likely to suddenly be content with accepting less.

The future generations of elderly will be used to using technological aids in the home-computer programmes, washing machines, televisions, videos, etc. etc., The transition to the use of technological aids to help them in their old age-emergency response systems-is therefore less ominous and would be reasonably easy for them. And the market is preparing to meet their needs.

What is more, in the particular situation of the Danish elderly population living in a welfare state it is quite clear from the results from the DaneAge Foundation's Future Study that the future generations of elderly in increasing numbers will be disinclined to allow themselves to be screened for public services-including emergency response systems. Therefore, a market is open. The future generations of elderly will also be willing to pay for these services and will certainly expect high quality services.

As far as technological aids in the home are concerned there would seem to be no imaginable limits. Perhaps Huxley's brave new world will turn into one which we could call the brave old (graying) world.

I have heard one or two things in the earlier papers of this symposium that have given me at least great cause for concern. For example the use of emergency response systems in the homes of working families where both parents are working and where we have what we in England call "latch key children" coming home to an empty house. And we are told, "Think of the security in having an emergency response system."

Now let's face it. What is wrong here is far too fundamental and profound to be solved by an emergency response system. It is a simple, unacceptable solution to a deep rooted social problem. And really we should be looking at these social problems. If we appear to solve them by providing technological aids, then I am sure that in time we will be creating even greater social problems. And social conditions that are eminently worthy of the harshest criticism would suddenly be acceptable. We must not accept them simply because we can install an emergency response system. We have to solve these profound problems.

And we have also heard about corporations worried about employees having to have time off to care for an elderly parent and therefor offering to have an emergency response system installed. Well how touching. Is an emergency response system really a solution there? It was Dylan Thomas who wrote:

Do not go gentle into that good night.
Old age should burn and rage at close of day.
Rage, rage against the dying of the light.

In an earlier intervention I responded to one of the speakers who was shocked because her mother, after a fall, had refused to have an emergency response system installed. Certainly one can fully understand the concern of the speaker in that situation living a great distance from her mother and feeling obviously unable to help. But are we providing false security? And, indeed, for whom are we providing this security? Is it really for the elderly person or is it for relatives or even the system? The worst thing we can do for elderly people is to deny them their denials of old age. In many cases it would probably be these denials that are keeping them going.

Finally, let me put to you one or two provocative questions in summary. What are we trying to achieve with emergency response systems? Are we trying to provide security, and if so, for whom? Are we trying to ally fears, and if so, for whom? Are we honestly doing it for the elderly? Or are we doing it for ourselves? For ourselves as relatives or for ourselves as the authorities, or indeed for ourselves as societies?

Is it because of a bad conscience that we develop emergency response systems, because I am sure I have heard earlier in the debate, that emergency response systems save only very few lives.

## LITERATURE

"Boliger" (Housing), Henrik Christoffersen and Leif Jakobsen, Copenhagen 1988.

"Befolkningen" (Population), George W. Leeson, P.C. Matthiessen and Hanne Spøhr, Copenhagen 1988.

"Politik" (Politics), Ole Borre, Copenhagen 1989.

"Holdninger og forventninger" (Attitudes and Expectations), Unni Bille-Brahe, Copenhagen 1989.

"Økonomi" (Economy), Thomas Mølsted Jørgensen, Copenhagen 1989.

"Helbred" (Health), Marianne Schroll, Copenhagen 1989.

"Service og informatik" (Services and Information), Oluf Danielsen, Copenhagen 1989.

"Arbejde og afgang" (Work and Retirement), Henning Friis, Copenhagen 1990.

"Fritid" (Leisure Time), Unni Bille-Brahe and Jørgen Bruun Pedersen, Copenhagen 1990.

"Older People and Technology-Policy and Practice," George W. Leeson, in "Older People and Technology," a report of Eurolink Age Seminar, Strasbourg, 1985.

"Two Way Communication Systems in Service for Older Citizens" experience from Denmark, Keld Møller, Paper presented at the 1st European Conference on The Bio-Tele Surveillance of Elderly People at Home, France, 1985.

"Nybyggeri og boligforsyning frem til år 2010" (New building and supply of housing till 2010), George W. Leeson (DaneAge Foundation) and Curt Liliegreen (The Danish Association of Contractors).

# Structure, Aims and Prospects of PRS in Germany

## Johannes Prass

In the following, a general description of the Emergency Response Service in the Federal Republic of Germany will be given as well as its structure, its aims and prospects. At the outset, the following remarks have to be made:

1. The Malteser-Hilfsdienst (Maltese Relief Organization) is a special association of German Caritas–a leading organization of voluntary welfare work in Germany–and as such it is intensively committed to the field of social services. The Emergency Response Service is one of the main responsibilities of the social work of the Malteser-Hilfsdienst. Not least this can also be seen in the fact that, today, the Malteser-Hilfsdienst, besides the German Red Cross, is the main supplier of Emergency Response Service in Germany. It has a network with more than 30 Emergency Response Centers and nearly 3,000 emergency call units.

The following description takes into account the rich experience and realization gained by the Malteser-Hilfsdienst during the many years of its commitment to Emergency Response Service; on the other hand, we will also describe the general situation of Emergency Response Service in the Federal Republic of Germany.

Johannes Prass is affiliated with Malteser-Hilfsdienst E.V., Germany.

2. Besides the demographic situation, technical equipment, financial conditions, etc., the main emphasis of this report will be put on the conception of the Emergency Response Service.

## DEMOGRAPHIC SITUATION AND DEVELOPMENT

At present, in the Federal Republic of Germany there are more than ten million people who are older than 65 years. According to estimates of the Federal Ministry for Young People, Families, Women and Health, we can assume that the increase in the total number of people about 65 will continue in the next years. Average life expectancy will increase and by the year 2000, will reach 67 years for men and 80 years for women. Especially the segment of aged people will considerably increase so that in the year 2000 about 2 million citizens will be older than 80, half a million will be older than 90 and about 10,000 older than 100 years.

At the same time, there is a drop in the birth rate. As a result, this fact leads to an increasing share of elderly people and a considerable alteration of the age diagram.

Another consequence is the increase in the need of care and attention. It is true that age on the one hand and need of care and attention on the other hand are not to be equated fundamentally; but nobody denies that increasing age also leads to an increasing number of people in need of care and attention.

Besides this numerical evolution, it is especially important for the significance of Emergency Response Service to recognize that elderly people increasingly wish to be personally independent and to remain in their usual domestic surroundings in their old age.

Therefore, further development of the social benefits system will be influenced by the realization that one main emphasis of help for the elderly people will be in the out-patient area. The establishment of further out-patient services takes into account the wish of most people in need of care and attention to live their life independently within their own four walls. Exaggerated care and attention may lead to the contrary of what is intended; i.e., to live an independent and dignified life. In this context, ERS offers to facilitate such an independent life. It also provides a respite for relatives and other caring persons.

## DEVELOPMENT OF EMERGENCY RESPONSE SERVICES IN THE FEDERAL REPUBLIC OF GERMANY

In the Federal Republic of Germany during the last ten years, a network of about 170 personal response centers has developed which has connected about 17,000 persons, most of whom are either elderly or handicapped. When putting these numbers in relation to the number of people over 65 in our country, one can certainly say that only an insignificantly small part of our elderly population up to now makes use of ERS.

Nevertheless, one can foresee an extensive development of ERS in the coming years. When looking at the last 10 years, one can note a considerable increase of subscribers to ERS, especially during the last two years, after ERS had to face enormous starting difficulties for many years. ERS was a totally new and unknown offer, and most elderly people to whom ERS was introduced had difficulty in accepting it, mostly due to their difficulty in accepting a mechanical device.

Over the years, we have succeeded, especially by means of well-directed public relations work of the supply organizations, in introducing the idea of ERS to the public. By having specific information in old people's homes and day centers and in doctor's practices, and by intensive personal advice, it was also possible to reduce people's inhibitions about ERS.

One can come to the conclusion that today ERS is not only known in the relevant target groups but also is absolutely accepted as a possible and potential emergency offer.

For the next years, the Malteser-Hilfsdienst and other supply organisations see their principal task in continuing to increase this degree of acceptance by means of intensive public relations work.

In this context, however, one should realize that, in many cases, costs for a connection to ERS are an obstacle for a subscription, despite the endeavors of the suppliers to keep them as low as possible. Certainly, one can be optimistic for the next years and hope that the public system of social benefits will increasingly support ERS in individual cases. In Section V more details will be given about this point.

## SUPPLY ORGANIZATIONS

In the Federal Republic of Germany, ERS is offered above all by charitable institutions and relief organizations and, in a few cases, by private organizations or councils and municipalities. Beside the German Red Cross, organizations of the Catholic and Protestant churches, i.e., Malteser-Hilfsdienst, Caritas, St. John's Ambulance and Diakonisches Werk, run most personal response centers.

On average, about 60 to 120 subscribers are connected to one personal response center. Beside small personal response centers, however, there are also big centers with more than 800 subscribers. According to the conception of ERS formulated by the Malteser-Hilfsdienst, a personal response center should not supply more than about 200 subscribers. The main argument for this restriction is the fact that otherwise individual care and service would not be ensured.

The increasing significance of ERS can also be seen in the fact that two umbrella organizations have been established which have made it their special business to promote and support ERS. One is the Working Group Communication Technology in the Federal Association of Voluntary Welfare Work (an amalgamation of the leading organizations of Voluntary Welfare Work in the Federal Republic of Germany). The other is the Federal Association of personal response services. The main tasks of these two institutions are public relations and representation of PRS interests with regard to public organizations and government ministries.

Besides those umbrella organisations, from time to time there is cooperation between several supply organisations of the same town. Altogether, one can say that there is sound competition between supply organisations; nevertheless, they generally subordinate their own interests to the wishes and requirements of frail persons.

## ORGANISATIONS AND TECHNICAL EQUIPMENT OF EMERGENCY RESPONSE SERVICE

From a technical point of view, Emergency Response Systems installed in Germany are a telecommunication system by means of which elderly, frail, sick or handicapped people, living alone in their home, can ask for specific help in emergency situations. This system consists of an Emergency Call Unit installed in the apartment of the frail person, the so-called FuFi mini-transmitter, a radio sensor which the subscriber can carry around his/her neck, and the Emergency Response Center which arranges the correct and proper help straight away. The emergency call, the acknowledgement of receipt and further signals are transmitted by the public telephone system of the Federal Post Office.

The Emergency Call Unit which consists of an emergency call button, a microphone and a loudspeaker is installed near the subscriber's telephone and connected to the telephone line. The Emergency Call Unit as well as the telephone should be put up in the apartment as centrally as possible. The home unit contains all necessary operating and indication elements as well as the electronics required for an automatic call to the Emergency Response Center by the telephone system for transmission of the emergency call, receipt and control signals. Besides the connection to the telephone system, one requires a connection to a socket. The microphone, which is integrated in the home unit, is activated only in case of an emergency, so that any disturbance of the private sphere or eavesdropping are completely impossible.

When the user presses the emergency call button, a voice connection between his apartment and the Emergency Response Center will be established in a matter of seconds. In certain emergency situations, the frail person may not be able to reach the emergency call button in the Emergency Call Unit. In these cases, the so-called FuFi transmitter, a small radio unit, will be of great help. This radio unit has a range of up to 150 meters to the Emergency Call Unit, depending on the local conditions. It is a small appliance which can be carried either in the pocket or around the neck by means of a hanger. When the emergency call is sent out by the radio unit, the integrated sender will transmit signals via a radio bridge to the Emergency Call Unit. Upon arrival of the emergency signals, dialing will be effected automatically. The emergency signals are transmitted to the Emergency Response Center. During this short period, the subscriber will hear an acoustic signal until the Center acknowledges receipt of the emergency call. By a loudspeaker which is integrated in the Emergency Call Unit contact can be established with a frail person. This intercom is technically so perfect that communication is possible from each corner of the apartment without using the receiver. In order to avoid acoustic feedbacks, the Emergency Response Center, by radio-control, turns the loudspeaker from speaking to hearing, from hearing to speaking.

For a great many elderly people, mainly elderly women, the previously quite large radio unit represented an essential argument against utilization of ERS. During the last few years, manufacturers not only technically optimized the radio unit but also reduced it to a size which corresponds to the size of a brooch.

Upon receipt of the emergency call, the Emergency Response Center immediately takes the necessary measures. Usually, the Emergency Response Center is installed in the same place where coordination and control of the emergency measures are effected. It is therefore often linked up with rescue situations. In order to ensure a high number of calls to be received by the telephone system, the Emergency Response Center normally has a private branch exchange with a unified telephone number and at least two telephone lines. Automatic switching in the Emergency Response Center ensures that, in case of several emergency calls, incoming at the same time, the Emergency Response Center remains obtainable by switching one of the lines to "free" immediately on receipt and acknowledgement of the emergency calls according to prescribed criteria of urgency. Should an Emergency Call Unit find the Emergency Response Center nevertheless busy, the Emergency Call Unit will finally reach the Emergency Response Center by means of automatic repetition of the dialing.

An emergency call incoming in the Emergency Response Center is analysed automatically with regard to the identity of the sender (numerically with digital indicator or EDP-visual display unit) and acknowledged immediately. Amongst those personal data are the following: name, place of residence, exact location of the apartment, age, possible diseases and handicaps, name, address and telephone number of the family doctor, names, addresses and telephone numbers of relatives and neighbors. If it is possible, the staff of the Emergency Response Center will first get a voice connection with the person seeking help in order to get to know more details about the emergency situation. Even if this is not possible, on the basis of the stored data it will be possible to arrange the required help for unconscious persons within a few minutes.

Neighbors and relatives who are prepared to help in case of emergency are an essential part of ERS; they should also have a key for the subscriber's apartment as they usually are the first persons to get into contact with the subscriber in case of emergency. Therefore, each subscriber, before being connected to the Emergency Response Center, should name at least four persons who are prepared to function as contacts. Many supply organisations help to find and to ask such persons.

Normally, the Emergency Response Centers are on duty around the clock, night and day. Due to the enormous need for staff, during the night smaller centers often join bigger ones without putting access at risk. Twenty four-hour access has proven to be an indispensible element of ERS; statistics show that many calls, especially real emergency calls, reach the Emergency Response Center either in the evening hours or in the early hours of the morning.


### FINANCING


#### *Costs for Suppliers and Manufacturers*


At present about ten manufacturers offer personal response centers, Emergency Call Units and accessories. Among these are very small firms exclusively manufacturing ERS appliances as well as worldwide companies conducting this branch of communication technology in specialized departments. The Malteser-Hilfsdienst collaborates exclusively with three German manufacturers. Because of competition, manufacturers are increasingly prepared to make concessions, especially when installing new ERS. These concessions may be considerable price reductions as well as the appointment of full-time assistants for after-sale-service.

Half of ERS costs for a new installation are covered by subsidies of the Lottery "Glucksspirale" (Wheel of Fortune) run by the German "Lottoblock." The remaining costs are covered by subsidies of councils and municipalities or by donations. New installation of PRS, despite the considerable investment costs, represents a minor financial problem compared to the running of the service which involves special financial charges mainly attributable to high personnel costs.

At the moment, costs for an Emergency Response Center range from DM 15,000 to DM 25,000, depending on size and equipment. Costs for an Emergency Call Unit range from DM 2,000 to DM 3,000. Although many manufacturers offer the possibility of leasing, supply organisations, as a rule, purchase Emergency Response Centers and Emergency Call Units; so the suppliers become owners of the Emergency Response Center and appliances.

Costs for a new installation of ERS therefore, on average, amount from about DM60,000 to 90,000 on the basis of 15 to 20 subscribers at the start.

*Costs for Suppliers and Subscribers*

Suppliers mostly rent appliances to subscribers, but are also increasingly offering the possibility of leasing or purchasing, especially for younger, handicapped persons.

The supply organization and subscriber conclude a contract arranging for rent for the equipment and maintenance and after-sale service by the supplier. It especially guarantees that emergency calls will be taken by the Emergency Response Centre, and that necessary help and assistance will be arranged straight away.

Monthly charges for the rent of the ERS appliances as well as maintenance and service by the personal response center at present are from DM 60 to 80 (Deutsche Mark). This charge does not include costs for a service alerted in case of emergency, e.g., doctor, rescue service, outpatient services or fire brigade, nor the installation costs of the Federal Post Office (at present DM 65), nor the current call charges of the subscriber. These costs have to be paid directly by the subscriber.

The majority of subscribers can bear the rental charges. However, in individual cases they may represent a strong financial burden and become an obstacle for subscription to ERS. If justified, suppliers grant a price reduction or do without payment of charges, however this cannot be generalized, and above all cannot be accepted as a solution of this problem.

The aid of public welfare institutions is needed since, up to now, they only contribute to the costs of ERS minimally. Health insurance as well as local institutions should give support in individual cases.

Up to now health insurance has generally declined to contribute to the costs of ERS. They do not recognize an Emergency Call Unit as a means of help in the sense of relevant prescriptions under the Health Insurance Law. This is regrettable since recognition of ERS as a means of help would mean a considerable financial saving for subscribers as well as for health insurers, at least when subscription to ERS would lead to a reduced stay in hospital.

In the future we must strive for a larger payment of subscribers' charges by resources of local public assistance institutions. The German Federal Public Assistance Law in several sections offers links for such payments, especially according to Section 75. In accordance with this section, elderly people must be helped in their old age. This assistance is aimed above all at preserving their independence and their participation in the life of society.

Another link of the Law could be Section 68 which provides for help for people in need of care and therefore may include the target group of subscribers to ERS.

Finally, it should be attempted to exempt telephone call charges for ERS. Up to now, however, proposals to this effect have always been rejected by the Federal Post Office.


## CONCEPTION OF ERS IN THEORY AND PRACTICE

If we look at ERS superficially, it may seem to be just a technical service providing help in the case of a possible but in practice comparatively seldom occurring medical emergency call. The essential concern of ERS, however, is the intensive social and psychosocial care of subscribers. To the church suppliers, the help of ERS is understood as an expression of real Christian brotherly love. Beside the possibility of arranging necessary help in emergency cases, ERS offers the possibility of telephone communication between the subscriber and the staff of the personal response center. Mostly, the calls are emotional calls for help, possibly concealed as test calls, expressing the wish for a short telephone conversation with the staff. These conversations essentially contribute to the emotional well-being of the concerned people and reduce risk in case of weak and delicate health. ERS gives the important feeling of being accepted by other people and of being needed and respected.

A subscriber once described it as follows: "If you feel lonely, you like to hear some friendly words, you do not need more." The 24 hour service and readiness for such conversations is an indispensable requirement of ERS as it is understood by Malteser-Hilfsdienst and other organizations.

Telephone contact is supplemented by intensive human contact and regular visits of ERS employees to the subscriber when there is time for conversation, a little help in daily tasks and perhaps even assistance and advice in difficult situations. These personal visits to the subscriber certainly make great demands on the organisational personnel; they are, however, an indispensable part of ERS.

Emergency Response services are not branches of the fire brigade or of rescue services, but an important part of the social net of outpatient services. ERS has equal value as other outpatient services and ideally should be offered in addition to them. In this way the ERS subscriber can be included in other services, e.g., "meals on wheels," transport services, neighbor help and other mobile social services. Possibly, the frail person will only get to know these outpatient services when subscribing to ERS.

In many towns the wealth of outpatient social services offered only permits "initiates" to have an overall picture of their range and their connections. The ERS employee who visits the subscriber at home should know the range of such services in the subscriber's catchment area and inform him or her about them.

Relatives under too great a strain due to care and attention may be released by ERS so that they can leave the house or even go on a journey free of worry.

In individual cases, the finding of new contacts might be an additional step to develop neighborly relations comprising tolerance and mutual assistance in emergency situations. When ERS was introduced about ten years ago, it was a main argument against this service to say that existing neighbor or family assistance would become unnecessary and would be destroyed. Today this reproach has not only been disproved, but it has also been found that ERS supports and strengthens social communication systems. Experience has shown that people previously unknown to the subscriber often are prepared to take responsibility as neighborly contacts for the subscriber in case of emergency.

It is certainly a task of supply organizations to be involved in the selection of such contacts. One should note that anxious, frail, old and overtaxed persons are not accepted as contact persons without reservation. Often a well directed search is necessary to find people who are glad to be able to help and who do not consider it just an obligation.

There are several reasons for suppliers to have qualified voluntary and full time staff:

a. The subscription of a person to ERS has to be combined with qualified consultation. The subscriber has not only to be informed about technical matters and financial charges; it is also very important to inspire confidence, to take the living situation into account, and to recognize possible needs and difficulties.

b. During a consultation on the occasion of the registration or cancellation of an Emergency Call Unit, important support can possibly be given to cope with changes, problems or losses. In many cases the Emergency Call Unit is disconnected due to removal of the person to an old people's home or a nursing home; during a conversation, the ERS employee can prepare for this step, and offer further assistance.

c. Cooperation with other social outpatient services often requires detailed knowledge about these services and their connections. Only on this basis is the ERS employee in a position to inform the subscriber on possible further help.

d. ERS often constitutes a link for people who are living alone and isolated, and who cannot come to meeting places of the parish or the community. On the occasion of the home visit the ERS employee may succeed in opening the elderly person step by step to social contacts. Besides human warmth and sensibility, this also demands a minimum of psychological and pedagogical knowledge.

## IN SUMMARY

The development of ERS as an offering in the outpatient services sector is based on the consideration that the proportion of elderly people in the total population has enormously increased during the last few years and will continue to increase until the year 2000. Besides the necessary inpatient institutions, it is absolutely necessary to offer outpatient services to meet the needs and requirements of elderly, sick and handicapped people. This is also intended by the legislative bodies which have established by law the priority of outpatient services.

ERS represents an important element of this general conception. One cannot do this without high quality standards. Furthermore, ERS must always be offered in connection with other outpatient social services.

# ISRAEL

# Emergency Response Systems in Israel

## David Cahn

### INTRODUCTION

This paper summarizes a survey commissioned by ESHEL and carried out by Megama Management and Planning Consultants in 1989.
The study surveyed equipment available in Israel and analyzed some 10 systems actually in use in 8 cities in Israel. Approximately 100 elderly persons and their relatives were interviewed in these cities. The aim of the survey and subsequent analysis was to provide state institutions, local authorities and the public in general with all the available information on existing systems, (which appeared in report form) on the state of the art, as well as supplying them with a users manual. This paper is based on those two publications.

### DEMOGRAPHIC INFORMATION

Emergency response services (ERS), are geared towards the elderly as a target population but they may also be useful for other populations such as the disabled, children or others.

David Cahn is affiliated with ESHEL.

In Israel, in 1987, the number of people over 65, in thousands, were as presented in Table 1.

The most recent detailed survey of all those over 65, carried out in 1985, including urban as well as rural populations, shows that of a total of 432,000, 22% were limited in their mobility.

The number of women over 65 living alone was three times that of men of the same age who lived alone. In 1985, 20% of all households owned by people over 70 were without a telephone. Of those over 65, 13% were childless and the children of another 3% lived abroad. Six per cent of the elderly had children who lived far from their parents' place of abode. The majority of the rest saw their parents frequently.

For the sake of analysis, the population was divided in four categories:

1. Those with medical problems. These were sub-divided as follows:

    1a. People living alone at high risk.
    1b. People at high risk.
    1c. People living alone, having a complicated medical history.
    1d. People with a complicated medical history.

2. People with medical problems requiring nursing care:

    2a. People living alone, disabled to various degrees, more or less bed-bound.
    2b. People disabled to various degrees, more or less bed-bound.
    2c. People in need of nursing care.

3. People at high security risk, living in a hostile environment.
4. Those interested in acquiring an alarm system for the sake of psychological assurance.

## TECHNOLOGY AND ORGANIZATION

The equipment surveyed was either available at time in Israel (1989), or in the development phase. Besides those manufactured locally, imported equipment was only considered if it was backed by local agents and servicing.

Certain basic features of any system were hypothesized. Thus:

    a. Alarm systems are to be deterrents and increase safety by discouraging would-be intruders.
    b. The most important function of any alarm system is to call for help.

Table 1   Population over age 65 (in thousands)

| Age | Total | Male | Female |
|-----|-------|------|--------|
| 65-69 | 125.1 | 58.9 | 66.2 |
| 70-74 | 106.4 | 47.6 | 58.8 |
| 75-79 | 88.1 | 41.4 | 46.7 |
| 80-84 | 44.3 | 21.0 | 23.3 |
| 85+ | 24.1 | 10.5 | 13.5 |
| Total | 388.0 | 179.4 | 208.5 |

The delivery of help can also vary. Help may come from outside: a relative, a base unit, a police station, the Magen David Adom (henceforth MDA), or any other organization. At the base unit there has to be immediate access to information on the caller, his state of health, where relatives may be reached, and where the key to his home is kept.

At times there may be a need for help with lesser degrees of urgency: callers may reach the police through pre-programmed codes on the phone, or contact the MDA the same way, or relatives who are "on call." Sometimes access to a willing conversation partner may be useful.

Help to be given at later points in time should also be considered: e.g., medical or nursing care, security calls, maintenance or social assistance.

Topography and physical environment must be taken into account in adapting systems to particular and local circumstances.

Alarm systems usually consist of four parts:

A home unit (the trigger), the alarm, the base unit and the responding agents.

The trigger may be fixed or mobile, telephone line or radio based. Signals and/or conversation may be one directional or two directional. There is a wide range of permutations possible based on these features.

It may be triggered through a button, movement in the room, lack of movement in the room, or by simply turning the system on.

The alarm system may be based on radio waves, laser or infrared waves, or voice frequency activation. The communication may be based on telephone cables, wireless or telephone lines with a wireless back-up system.

The operation of alarm systems must be easy for the user.

Here are some guidelines on the ergonomics of personal units:

- Size and weight must be low.
- The trigger of the home unit must be such that the caller has to be able to hang it around his neck, or attach it to his wrist or his belt.

- If it is water and shatter-proof, the likelihood of break-down decreases.
- Operation must be simple, taking into account that at moments of crisis a one-stage operation is warranted.
- The button or trigger itself must be easy to access and to activate.
- It is useful if a feed-back is there for the caller to know that he has effected the call.

In short, the home unit must not be cumbersome.

Some routine of checks must ascertain that the system is on. Daily tests are recommended.

The two most important features of any system are dependability and resilience. The fewer the number of components and the higher their quality, the most likely it is that this can be achieved. The more simple a unit, the more dependable it will be.

A system may be able to provide services in addition to the ones discussed above. Thus, it may be used as a general alarm (siren), smoke-detector, or detector of gas leaks. A secondary set of subscribers may also be given service.

Like the home unit, the base unit may also be phone or wireless based. It may be fixed, mobile or part of a network. Callers' data must be accessible to personnel at the base unit. Computerized systems give ample information on the caller (his condition, accessibility, relatives, etc.). Special equipment may convey the call directly to agents able to help and also be able to cancel the call.

The equipment may be obtained through various arrangements. It may be purchased or rented. The services may be provided with a monthly or periodical payment or to be paid as used, i.e., for each call.

### The Technological Equipment Available in Israel

One may say that most equipment available in the world is also available in Israel. Local manufacturers, however, enjoy some preference, mostly because they are able to provide back-up and service.

Foreign manufacturers with local agents are next on the list of preference, provided they can offer service.

Some of the Israeli manufacturers supply parts for the other manufacturers' systems.

Israeli companies may be classified thus:

1. Calls using telephone infrastructure: Visonic, Electronics Line, Aminut, Gil-Ad, Secutec, Kol Adir, Bezek, Telrad and some other 20 companies.

2. Alarm calls through radio transmitters: Motorola, Ofer Shapid (representing Homelink), Superviser and another five companies.
3. Nationwide systems are "Yad Sarah" and "Secutec."
4. Security services are provided by: "Hashomer Israel," "Hashmira, Moked 99," "Agudath Hashmira" and many others.
5. Some of the networks providing alarm services are: "Ramid" (representing "Tetco"), "Visonic" and "Motorola," "Ofer Shapir," "Beeper," "Aminut" and "Iturit."

*Evaluation of Available Systems*

There are some general grounds for evaluation. The following table (Table 2) sums up the survey's findings and recommendations:

It is possible to conclude that since there are no major differences between the equipment of the various companies surveyed, companies which have been around for longer are more likely to be reliable having accumulated experience in use of equipment.

Generally, telephone based systems are preferable to the wireless type. Telephones are to be found in many homes. Their operation is simpler, telephones break down less frequently, and the telephone company's maintenance infrastructure may serve the alarm system as well.

The following table (Table 3) sums up the efficiency of the systems surveyed. It considers, in addition to cost of purchase, running costs, reliability and service. A simple scale from one to three is used to assess systems; one being for the most recommended system while three for the least recommended.

It is useful to list the organizations in Israel concerned with the elderly.

• MDA have someone on duty around the clock and have stations scattered throughout the entire country. They respond efficiently and reliably. They do not have extra resources but there is the possibility that another body could cover the costs of developing a network for emergency calls.

• The police and the Civil Guard can be considered as they too have bases scattered around the country. They are reliable and efficient but also have some disadvantages: there can conceivably be situations when no immediate response can be expected as there might be some other prior emergency.

• "Kuppath Holim" (the sick fund) has a nationwide infrastructure and its personnel are qualified and able to give the best of help but only at hours that the clinics are open.

- "Yad Sarah," a voluntary organization, is already operating a system with a base unit in Jerusalem. "Yad Sarah" has been the first organization in Israel to set up and run an ERS. It plans to set up an additional network for the rest of the country. The Jerusalem system has a maximum capacity of 10,000 elderly. "Yad Sarah" intends to run its nationwide ERS with a computerized headquarters, and the 60 branches it has would serve as infrastructure.
- Local authorities are also concerned with the elderly. They are receptive to the subject of ERS.
- "Amidar," a government housing corporation, is "landlord" to some 27,000 citizens over 65 who rent flats from it. The company lists high amongst its priorities the subject of services to the elderly in their homes. Amidar has a certain amount of financial resources it could channel to ERS.
- Community Centers, "Matnasim," are scattered around the country, some 150 in number. They are in a position to cooperate organizationally provided funding is forthcoming from other sources.
- "Bezek," the telephone company, is about to institute a service which should be triggered 20 seconds after the phone is off the hook and no number has been dialed. This will automatically connect the number to an operator who will be able to listen to what happens in the room and summon help if necessary.

Possible sources of finance for ERS are:

- "Eshel" is the organization in charge of planning and developing services for the elderly in Israel. It can participate in paying for the setting up of an ERS and can even provide professional personnel.
- The National Insurance Institute, NII, will provide a budget for those elderly eligible for assistance under the new Nursing Care Law. It can further provide consumer guidance to the elderly when they are faced with a choice between the various systems.
- The Ministry of labor and Social Welfare, can also fund some of the expenses involved as it has a portion of its budget earmarked to serve the elderly.
- "The Council for the Aged" can also provide some financial support through funds it raises such as via the "Teletrom" which is a marathon TV fundraising campaign.
- "Project Renewal," an urban renewal program, can also provide certain resources. This would have to be specifically for the elderly within the neighborhood they are responsible for.

- Finally, voluntary organizations such as the Rotary Club, may contribute financial assistance in individual cases they approve.

There is potential for the ERS in the private sector. Some 300 companies already provide security services. They operate base units and can provide their subscribers with wireless or telephone operated home units, which they may supply to individual users, sponsoring institutions or to non-profit organizations. There is one company currently planning a nationwide network of ERS.

## COST OF EQUIPMENT AND SERVICE PER PERSON

Individual home units cost least in the case when base units already exist. In considering the cost of adding a new user to an existing system, we may disregard the cost of initial capital investments in setting up the system itself.

Based on the sample of the survey, to join a wireless system the cost ranges from the most expensive (in Yahud), $1,773, to the cheapest (in Rehovoth), $926. To join a telephone based system the cost ranges from (Petah Tiquvah), $1.314, to the lowest cost (in Rehovoth) at $651. The difference in cost between wireless and telephone-based systems reflects the fact that in the case of the former, here is no need to buy equipment. The cost is lowest in the case of mobile base unit, i.e., only $300.

When doing a cost analysis, it is necessary to take into account the payment scheme. For example, though $1,685. (in Ashdod) might seem high, as a lump sum, if we distribute payment over ten years, at $20 a month, it seems more reasonable.

## CRITERIA FOR A PERSON TO BE INCLUDED
## IN COVERAGE PLAN

The majority of users of ERS are elderly people living alone, afraid of possible medical emergency, assuming that they would be unable to call for help the ordinary way.

In the survey on which this report is based, the following categories of need for ERS were analyzed:

Table 2.  Evaluation of Alarm Systems

| TYPE | ADVANTAGES | DISADVANTAGES | LIMITATIONS |
|------|-----------|---------------|-------------|
| tele- phoen based | * lower cost<br>* available<br>* easy use<br>* modular<br>* multiple<br>help agents<br>may be reached | * faults in line<br>* lines overload<br>* no reply | * 100 calls<br>* lines overload<br>* installation<br>lengthy |
| wireless based | * may be used<br>anywhere | * costly<br>* transmitter<br>disturbances?<br>* only specific<br>help may be<br>summoned.<br>* no answer?<br>* equipment heavy<br>and cumbersome. | * physical en-<br>vironment<br>(e.g. moun-<br>tains, etc.) |
| fixed based unit sending pat- rol or other form of help | * human interac-<br>tion<br>* qualifications | * human reaction-<br>may be delayed<br>resources<br>may be inadequate | *limitations<br>of human |
| mobile base units (network) | * lower cost<br>* personal<br>acquaintance<br>with sub-<br>scriber | usually manned by<br>volunteers<br>* limited phy-<br>sical area | limited to<br>communities<br>or small<br>neighbour-<br>hoods |

Table 3   Ratings of Alarm Systems

| Possible types | Territory | Efficiency | Reliability | Service |
|---|---|---|---|---|
| * 'phone based with fixed base unit | urban | 1 | 3 | very good |
| * 'phone based with mobile base unit | urban | 2 | 1 | good |
| Possible types | Territory | Efficiency | Reliability | Service |
| *mixed, ( 'phone and wire-less based) with fixed base unit | urban | 2 | 2 | good |
| *wire-less network+ mobile base unit | communal | 1 | 1 | mediocre |

- High medical risk + living alone ............................ 20%
- High medical risk ............................................... 12%
- Those with a complicated medical history ................ 18%
- Disability + bedriddenness + living alone ............... 11%
- In need of nursing care ........................................ 9%
- Security risk ...................................................... 4%
- No special need (except psychological) ................... 26%

From this list it would appear that about 50% are at high medical risk or have a complicated medical history. Paradoxically there is an inverse relationship between the extent to which a person needs access to an ERS, the mental and/or physical ability to make use of it and the means to pay for it. In order to identify the population likely to benefit from ERS it is recommended to consider a wide population. When deciding who, from among that population, should receive subsidy, the focus may be narrowed.

## OPERATIONS AND USE

The elderly who were interviewed made very low use of the alarm system. Each user, on average, made between 1/2 to 3 calls per year. The users were mostly old people living alone. They subscribed to an ERS for fear of not being able to call for help at a time of medical or security emergency unless, as in the case of an ERS, they only needed to push a button.

Though many disabled people find ERS most useful, it must be noted that most systems are not designed to meet nursing care needs. One of the limitations of most systems is that they lack the flexibility to accommodate individual needs of subscribers (e.g., the case of a blind user who was interviewed and who had been supplied a fixed trigger on a wall though he would have been far better served by a mobile one).

Emergencies are clearly more frequently of medical rather than security problems. Sixty percent of users interviewed said they feared medical emergencies and only 20% were worried about safety or security. Ninety percent of calls actually were for medical emergencies.

In general, the number of calls made is very low. There were some false alarms. There is disagreement between users, who usually claim not to have triggered a call, and attendants who do not believe the call was a dysfunction of the system. One of the unintended consequences of the low frequency of use is that there is insufficient knowledge of the functional level of the system.

As regards users' resistance, barriers to use, and user satisfaction, the following was found:

Triggers are most often located near the bed. In the case of bedridden users, the reason is obvious but even users who are mobile are suspicious of mobile triggers, fearing that they are too sensitive to touch and may increase the frequency of false alarms.

There is little knowledge of the technological or the human sides of the system. Because of the characteristics of the users, even a higher level of understanding is no guarantee that at a time of crisis this understanding would not falter. There were some reports of interviewees complaining of not having been well enough instructed or of having forgotten the instructions received when the home unit was affixed.

Some users felt that the system is alien and alienating because of its technological level which is above the one they were used to.

The systems surveyed all had one-way communications. Likewise, most home units were fixed. It was reported at times of real emergency one user was unable to make the call as he was not near the trigger. No case was reported of users initiating a call in order to test the system.

## BENEFITS AND FAULTS OF ERS

Users claimed the system had no influence on their daily lives. Generally old people were pleased, however, to know that a trigger has been installed in their house and hoped not to have to use it.

It seems that the system's main positive but unintended consequence is the peace of mind it provides and this is important for the user and his family. On the other hand, no negative consequences were found, such as a decline of attention relatives had been giving the elderly prior to joining the alarm system.

It should be noted here that an ERS only meets the extreme needs of the elderly while their daily needs must be met by other services. Since this is a population reluctant to make demands and one not sufficiently aware of their rights, care must be taken that a sense of complacency on behalf of those responsible, does not set in on account of an ERS having been installed.

Though in principle the ERS is designed to offer immediate emergency relief, it is necessary to follow up through the health and welfare system. For that purpose, every call should be reported daily to the pertinent authorities responsible for the subject's health. In case of hospitalization, relatives must be informed immediately.

The existence of a body responsible for an alarm system for the elderly can be the basis for providing additional services in that particular location. Examples are: increased security arrangements and support for the elderly. These, however, are secondary benefits while the main ones are, as stated above, peace of mind for users and their relatives.

A number of faults were identified:

a. None of the systems in the survey were used to their full potential. (they served only 30-300 subscribers out of a potential of thousands).
b. Users are not trained fully to benefit from their systems.
c. Maintenance is not always at optimal level.
d. The check-up system is not operational.

Despite all that, users are generally satisfied with the system they subscribe to. ERS thus has a positive influence on the sense of security of the users, fears are greatly mitigated and in more than one case, ERS has saved human life.

It is also possible to project that when the carrying capacity of the systems is fully utilized, all other services pertinent to the elderly will be affected. The visibility of an otherwise silent population will improve, and with it, it is to be expected, their voices will become more audible and therefore their overall medical and social rights will be better met.

Return on investment in ERS is to be expected to be high. Early attention to medical problems can avoid lengthy hospitalization and costly medical treatment, on the one hand, while, on the other, the cost of dispatching ambulance services when this is not necessary can be avoided.

One can further extrapolate from the data obtained in the survey that as the number of subscribers will increase, the cost, per head, will decrease dramatically.

## EXPECTED FUTURE DEVELOPMENTS

It has been found that one of the most consistent shortcomings of existing systems surveyed has been their inability for two-way communication. It is to be welcomed, therefore, that the trend of manufacturers everywhere has been to incorporate such a feature in future systems.

In Israel specifically, the new trends are, on an organizational level, to set up national systems as opposed to the local ones operating. The economic benefits to be expected are a lowering of costs per user, through "economies of scale" while, at the same time, the hardware itself is being manufactured at lower costs all the time. So, in short, it is possible to look forward to a definite decrease in cost per user.

Finally, at the risk of reiteration, it may be added that the most important points made here have been the already existing capacity of ERS to save human life, which is of importance beyond anything else that could be said. If, in addition, peace of mind and increased quality of life is attained, any future improvement would be blessing upon blessing.

We should always remember, however, that any technologically based system is only as intelligent and as kind as its human component and that no amount of technological advance should allow us to lose sight of that fact.

# JAPAN

# Recent Trends of ERS in Japan

## Masayuki Abe

### OVERVIEW OF ERS IN JAPAN

#### The Aging of Society

*Aging of Population*

The elderly population (65 years and older) of Japan was 13,785,000 as of 1988, constituting 11.2% of the total population of 122,783,000 (Table 1).

The substantial increase in Japan's elderly population is expected to continue in the future, with the figure reaching 12,338,000 in the year 2000. This will be 16.3% of the total population, which is about the level of that in Western countries at present.

Moreover, in 2021, when the ratio of elderly population reaches its first peak, the figure will be 31,866,000, making up about 23.6% of the total. This will mean the arrival of a society with a higher ratio of elderly persons than any other country has so far experienced (see Figure 1).

#### Changes in Family Environment

*Increase in Aged Households.* The trend in Japan's households has been continuing towards the nuclear family since the end of World War II. The

Masayuki Abe is affiliated with Nippon Telegraph and Telephone Corporation, Japan.

TABLE 1:  TRANSITION OF ELDERLY POPULATION

(Unit:  Thousand People; %)

| Year | Population | | | Ratio to Total Population | |
|------|-----------|---|---|---|---|
| | Total Population | 65 Years and Older | 75 Years and Older | 65 Years and Older | 75 Years and Older |
| 1960 | 94,032 | 5,398 | 1,642 | 5.7 | 1.7 |
| 1965 | 99,209 | 6,236 | 1,894 | 6.3 | 1.9 |
| 1975 | 111,940 | 8,865 | 2,841 | 7.9 | 2.5 |
| 1985 | 121,049 | 12,468 | 4,712 | 10.3 | 3.9 |
| 1988 | 22,783 | 13,785 | 5,479 | 11.2 | 4.5 |
| 1990 | 124,224 | 14,819 | 5,917 | 11.9 | 4.8 |
| 2000 | 131,192 | 21,338 | 8,452 | 16.3 | 6.4 |
| 2010 | 135,823 | 27,104 | 12,456 | 20.04 | 9.2 |
| 2020 | 135,304 | 31,880 | 15,313 | 23.56 | 11.3 |
| 2021 | 135,160 | 31,866 | 15,239 | 23.58 | 11.3 |
| 2025 | 134,642 | 31,465 | 17,367 | 23.4 | 12.9 |

(Source:)      "National Census" by Statistics Bureau of Management and Coordination Agency;
"Japan's Future Population" by the Institute of Population Issues, Ministry
of Health and Welfare.

average number of family members was 5.00 persons in 1953, 3.75 persons in 1965, and reached 3.19 persons in 1987 (Table 2). Under these circumstances, the increase in the number of aged households has been remarkable. This number has gone up from 799,000 in 1965, 1,619,000 in 1975, to 3,731,000 in 1988. This is 4.7 times larger than the figure for 1965, and substantially exceeds the growth in general households.

*Increase in Elderly People Living Alone.* As the elderly get older, they come to live alone with the death of their spouses and for other reasons. In

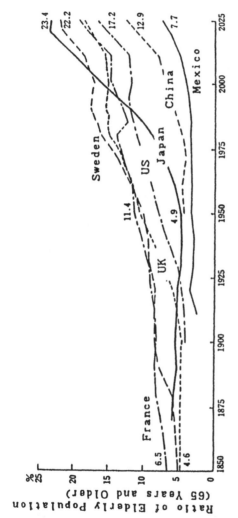

FIGURE 1: TRANSITION OF POPULATION RATIOS FOR 65 YEARS AND OLDER
IN MAJOR COUNTRIES

Source: "National Census" by Statistics Bureau of Management and
Coordination Agency and "Japan's Future Population" by the
Institute of Population Issues, Ministry of Health and Welfare for
Japan; and UN "Population Studies" for other countries.

TABLE 2: YEARLY TRANSITION IN TOTAL AND AGED HOUSEHOLDS

| Year | Number of Total Households | | | Number of Aged Households | | $\dfrac{(B)}{(A)}$ × 100 |
|---|---|---|---|---|---|---|
| | Estimated (1,000 Households) (A) | Index (1965 = 100) | Average Household Size (Persons) | Estimated (1,000 Households) (B) | Index (1965 = 100) | |
| 1953 | 17,180 | 66 | 5.00 | 431 | 54 | 2.5 |
| 1955 | 18,963 | 73 | 4.68 | 425 | 53 | 2.2 |
| 1960 | 22,476 | 87 | 4.13 | 500 | 63 | 2.2 |
| 1965 | 25,940 | 100 | 3.75 | 799 | 100 | 3.1 |
| 1970 | 29.887 | 115 | 3.45 | 1,196 | 150 | 4.0 |
| 1975 | 32,877 | 127 | 3.35 | 1,619 | 203 | 4.9 |
| 1980 | 35,333 | 136 | 3.28 | 2,424 | 303 | 6.9 |
| 1985 | 37,226 | 144 | 3.22 | 3,110 | 389 | 8.4 |
| 1986 | 37,544 | 145 | 3.22 | 3,320 | 416 | 8.8 |
| 1987 | 38,064 | 147 | 3.19 | 3,471 | 434 | 9.1 |
| 1988 | 39,028 | 150 | 3.12 | 3,731 | 467 | 9.6 |

(Source:) "Basic Research of Welfare Administration" and "Basic Research of National Life," both issued by the Statistics Information Division of Ministry of Health and Welfare.

1973, there were 578,000 elderly people living alone, accounting for 6.8% of the over-65 population (Table 3). This ratio has been rising year by year and by 1988 constituted 1,405,000 people, or 10.4% of the aged population.

According to future estimates for older people living alone, it is believed the number will continue to increase drastically, up to 2,440,000 in the year 2000 and 3,983,000 in 2025.

TABLE 3: YEARLY TOTALS OF ELDERLY PEOPLE LIVING ALONE

(Unit: Thousand People; 5)

| Year | Over-65 Population | Number of | Elderly | Living Alone | Ratio of Elderly Living Alone [(B)/(A)] |
|------|------|------|------|------|------|
| | | Total (B) | Male | Female | |
| 1973 | 8,466 | 578 | - | - | 6.8 |
| 1978 | 9,921 | 754 | 164 | 590 | 7.6 |
| 1980 | 10,729 | 910 | 192 | 718 | 8.5 |
| 1981 | 11,117 | 984 | 200 | 784 | 8.9 |
| 1982 | 11,515 | 976 | 222 | 754 | 8.5 |
| 1983 | 11,486 | 1,046 | 216 | 830 | 9.1 |
| 1984 | 11,718 | 1,147 | 240 | 907 | 9.8 |
| 1985 | 12,111 | 1,131 | 218 | 913 | 9.3 |
| 1986 | 12,626 | 1,281 | - | - | 10.1 |
| 1987 | 13,030 | 1,290 | 242 | 1,048 | 9.9 |
| 1988 | 13,491 | 1,405 | 286 | 1,119 | 10.4 |

(Source:) "Basic research of Welfare Administration" and "Basic Research of National Life," both issued by the Statistics Information Division of Ministry of health and Welfare.

## ERS Overview

Various problems of the aging society have begun to be apparent since 1975. Among them, a major topic was the problem of elderly people living alone, particularly those in poor health who were found to be living in insecure conditions as they had no way to deal with emergencies such as sudden illness and accident. The ERS introduced by Tokyo's Musashino Welfare Public Corporation in 1981 is considered to be the beginning of

ERS in Japan. Following this, other municipalities and private businesses also started to provide ERS, thus expanding ERS coverage.

However, the history of ERS in Japan is still young, as it was just a few years ago that it was introduced in earnest. Therefore, about 26,000 people, or only 2% of the elderly living alone, are using ERS as of the end of fiscal 1989.

## Service Overview

Essentially, there are no major differences between public and private ERS, all of which provide the following basic service: When elderly people living alone face emergencies such as illness or accident at home:

1. Pushing the emergency button on a pendant radio transmitter worn by the aged person automatically sends a telephone signal to an ERS center which is manned on a 24-hour basis.
2. Once the center receives a signal, a computer produces a CRT display of previously registered user data (name, address, past illness, contact persons, etc.).
3. Operators at the center confirm the user's situation by telephone or ask contact persons to confirm the situation. In case of emergency, the center requests the dispatch of an ambulance, fire engine or police.

## ERS as Administrative Welfare Service

*Present Situation of ERS Introduction.* According to a 1988 survey by the Ministry of Home Affairs and the Fire Defense Agency, about 230 of the nation's 3,200 municipalities have introduced ERS since its introduction by Tokyo's Musashino Welfare Public Corporation. Although no actual statistics are available, the number of the nation's elderly users living alone is estimated at about 20,000.

## People Involved in ERS Operation

1. *Operators of ERS Center.* Because of the need to provide 24-hour service, the operation is carried out by fire department headquarters in many cases. In other cases, the operation is entrusted to local emergency centers, or private companies.
2. *Contact Persons.* Three or four contact persons, such as local welfare officers or neighbors on a volunteer basis, are required to go to

the home of an elderly person living alone and confirm the situation in case of emergency.

3. *Fire Stations for the Dispatch of Ambulances, etc.*

*ERS Target Users.* While there are some minor differences among municipalities, target users are mostly low-income people living alone, who are either over 65 or are seriously disabled.

*ERS Cost Structure.* As with target users, there are some differences among municipalities. Generally, however, the cost of installing the equipment and the rental fee without telephone charges is free for the target users.

The cost of equipment, installation costs and operational costs are paid by local governments.

*ERS Promotion by National Government.* As a national measure, the Ministry of Health and Welfare, the Ministry of Home Affairs and the Fire Defense Agency began to financially support the introduction of ERS by local governments one or two years ago, and are promoting the expansion of ERS throughout the country.

The Ministry of Health and Welfare is planning to financially assist 330 municipalities during the five years from fiscal 1988, while the Ministry of Home Affairs and the Fire Defense Agency are planning to support 50 municipalities during the three years from fiscal 1989.

## ERS as Private Business Operations

*Introduction of ERS by Private Companies.* In the private sector, a security firm started providing ERS to ordinary households in 1982, as an addition to the many home-security services. Presently, a number of companies in the medical service industry, private retirement homes and taxi companies, as well as security firms, are offering ERS as part of management diversification strategies.

Based on newspaper and magazine information, we estimate that there are dozens of private companies that are offering ERS. Among them, one or two companies are thought to specialize in ERS.

There are about 6,000 people using private ERS.

*Number of Employees.* The number of employees engaged in ERS operations ranges from five to 30 per company. Thus it is still small in terms of scale.

*Service Area.* In most cases, ERS coverage is limited to within prefectural boundaries.

*Charges.* Charges to members consist of an enrollment fee, installation fee, and charges for use. In general, the enrollment fee is 30,000 ($200), the installation fee is 10,000 ($66), and the equipment rental charge is 3,000 ($20) (dollar conversion rate of $1/150).

*Membership.* One company is said to be providing service to 1,000 members, but the average membership is about 300.

## OUTLINE OF MOST COMMON ERS EQUIPMENT

ERS equipment can roughly be classified into two types of equipment: ERS user equipment for people living alone and ERS center equipment.

Companies supplying such equipment are mainly NTT and makers of communications equipment (see Photo). The leading companies are estimated to be about ten or more.

There is little difference in price or functions of ERS equipment offered by various companies. ERS user equipment, which consists of a pendant radio transmitter and a telephone, costs about 10,000 ($667). ERS center equipment (including software) costs about 3 million ($20,000), and consists of personal computers, emergency signal receiving equipment, etc.

Typical equipment and the functions of each are outlined below.

### ERS User Equipment

As illustrated in Figure 2, ERS user equipment consists of a pendant radio transmitter and a telephone set for emergency signal transmission. When elderly persons living alone are faced by an emergency such as sudden illness or accident, they push a button on the pendant and the ERS equipment automatically sends a signal to the ERS center.

ERS user equipment is composed of the basic units ((1) - (3), (7)) and option units ((4) - (6)).

*Pendant Radio Transmitter (1).* Users always wear the pendant radio transmitter, and push the button on the transmitter in an emergency, thus transmitting a radio signal.

The pendant button is designed to be pushed easily in a one-touch operation. The radio signal emitted is effective within the range of 20 meters from a radio receiver. Since it is very important that the transmitter can be used within a toilet or bathroom, a radio transmission test is always conducted at the time of installation.

*Radio Receiver (2).* A radio receiver receives the signal from the pendant transmitter and sends it to the telephone set.

*Telephone Set for Emergency Signal Transmission (3).* This telephone set receives the signal front the radio receiver, automatically dials the number of the ERS center where the user's name is registered, and also transmits the ID of the user.

PHOTO: NIT Equipment in Emergency Response Center.

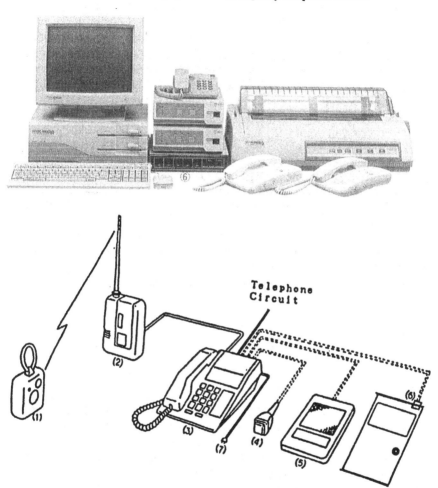

FIGURE 2: ERS USER EQUIPMENT LINEUP

*Remote Switch (4).* A remote switch is connected with the telephone set via wire for emergency signal transmission. A user places the remote switch next to the pillow or somewhere convenient, and pushes the button in an emergency.

*Hands-Free Speaker (5).* This automatic-response equipment is connected to the telephone set, and permits the user to talk to the operator at the ERS center without picking up the telephone handset. From a structural standpoint, it is effective within a range of five meters.

*Sensor (6)*. This device is installed on a toilet door, for example, to monitor whether a user opens and closes the door within fixed periods of time, and automatically reports the results to the ERS center. If the door isn't opened or closed, the ERS center contacts the user for confirmation.

*Commercial Power Source (7)*. The telephone set for emergency signal transmission, radio receiver and hands-free speaker are operated by a commercial power source. In the event of outage, however, up to about six-hours of operation is possible by the built-in battery.

### ERS Center Equipment

ERS center equipment consists of personal computers and emergency signal receiving units. The names and addresses of users and the telephone numbers of their contact persons (local welfare officers and neighbors) are stored in a database on the personal compute disk. This information is updated as required.

When a user's ID is received through the telephone line by the emergency signal receiving unit, the personal computer retrieves the database information for the user and displays it on the screen. Based on this information, center operators confirm the user's condition or call the contact persons or a fire station.

## SPECIFIC EXAMPLES OF ERS IN JAPAN

### Kashiwa City's ERS

Kashiwa City is located 70 kilometers east of Tokyo, and covers an area of about 73 square kilometers. It is an area that has seen remarkable development recently as a bed-town community.

The Kashiwa City's ERS started service in December 1989, targeting elderly people living alone in the city as an administrative welfare service with the fire department headquarters as the reception center. This format of carrying out ERS on a municipal-unit basis and installing the ERS reception center in the fire department headquarters is the most common type of operation in Japan.

### Service Features

As the fire department headquarters is assigned as the ERS reception center, it meets all the requirements of an ERS center mentioned below, thus being most appropriate to save the lives of enfeebled persons in case of emergency.

1. Able to respond promptly in case of emergency, on a 24-hour basis.
2. Able to secure a certain number of personnel who can take action immediately.
3. Defined direction and order system, with clear-cut lines of responsibility. Moreover, the center dispatches an ambulance immediately on receipt of a signal if a user does not respond to a call from the center.

## Target Users

1. Elderly people 65 and older living alone in the city. As of February 1990, 18 people are using the service. There are 1,100 elderly people living alone, making a diffusion rate of 1.6%.
2. Disabled people living alone. So far, there were no users as of February 1990.

## ERS Reception Situation (December 1989-February 1990)

The reception situation is shown in Table 4.

TABLE 4: KASHIWA CITY'S ERS RECEPTION SITUATION

| Total Signals Received | 16 | |
|---|---|---|
| Reception Contents | | |
| Request for Help | 0 | |
| Counseling | 2 (13%) | Informed Contact Person |
| Checking if Really Connected | 3 (19%) | |
| Pushed Pendant Button in Error | 4 (25%) | |
| Unplugged from Power Source | 7 (43%) | |

*Contact Persons*

Three contact persons are registered for each user. (One of the three is a local welfare officer.)

*Cost Structure*

The cost of ERS user equipment (about 100,000 ($667)) is fully paid by the city. Users pay telephone call charges.

*Items to Be Improved*

In proceeding with user expansion in the future, it will be difficult to secure contact persons. Especially, as there are few people who want to become welfare officers, they will be responsible for plural uses which will increase the burden on them.

## Miyagi Prefecture's ERS

Miyagi Prefecture is located 250 kilometers northeast of Tokyo. The prefecture is about 7,300 square kilometers in area, and includes 71 municipalities within a 70-km radius of Sendai City.

Miyagi Prefecture's ERS started as an administrative welfare service in August 1988. This is unique type of operation in Japan with respect to the fact that it covers municipalities throughout the prefecture and the ERS center in Sendai City is operated by a medical-related organization.

*Service Features*

1. In June 1988, Miyagi Prefecture entrusted the operations of the ERS center to the Miyagi Prefecture Local Medical Information Center Foundation, which was jointly established by the Miyagi Prefecture and the Miyagi Prefecture Medical Association.

The center combines various kinds of information, such as information on types of hospitals, infectious diseases and medical examination information in its 24-hour system. And because the communications system connecting the ERS center with the fire department headquarters and medical institutions is established as a medical information network, system cooperation enables people to promptly deal with emergencies such as hospitalization.

2. Since only one ERS center is providing service for all municipalities in Miyagi Prefecture, the costs to be borne by each municipality involve only those of ERS user equipment, and do not include the installation and personnel costs that each municipality would face if it were to establish its own ERS center. This makes system expansion easier.

3. Sensors attached to the toilet or kitchen door automatically transmit to the ERS center once a day data on whether the doors have been opened or not, thereby permitting early discovery if users are unable to move because of sudden illness or death.

*Target Users*

1. Elderly people in the prefecture who are 65 years or older and living alone. As of February 1990, 35 municipalities (out of 71) in Miyagi Prefecture had joined and the service covers 700 users. The number of aged people living alone in Miyagi Prefecture is about 10,000, or a diffusion rate of 7.5%.

2. Disabled people in the prefecture who are living alone. As of February 1990, there were 15 users (Tables 5 and 6).

*ERS Reception Situation (April 1989-February 1990)*

*Contact Persons*

Three contact persons are registered for each user (one of the three is a local welfare officer).

*Cost Structure*

The cost of ERS user equipment (about 100,000 ($667)) is fully paid by the national government (Ministry of Health and Welfare), the prefecture, or the municipality. Users pay telephone call charges.

*Items to Be Improved*

1. To expand the coverage area where service is to be introduced (scheduled to cover all municipalities in the prefecture by the end of

March 1993; users estimated at about 2,250), it is necessary to increase personnel at the ERS center and to expand facilities.

2. Constant monitoring is conducted by sensor, but it is necessary to improve ERS user equipment in order to reduce troublesome handling of signals both by users and the center.

## Safety Center's ERS

As a private business, the Safety Center's ERS started in Tokyo in December 1987 to specialize in this service targeted on elderly people living alone, throughout the country. As it targets the whole country, it has installed sub-centers in local areas. There are also participating users in Hokkaido, which is 1,000 kilometers away from Tokyo.

## Safety Features

1. Personnel with nursing qualifications are on duty on a 24-hour basis.
2. By keeping in touch with the contact person to confirm the situation, ambulance dispatch requests are kept to the lowest necessary level.
3. Selling points include attentive service including various consultations.

TABLE 5:     MIYAGI PREFECTURE'S ERS RECEPTION SITUATION (1/2) (Emergency Button Pushed or

Abnormality in Power Source)

| | | |
|---|---|---|
| Total Signals received | 443 | |
| Reception Contents | | |
| (1) Request for Help | 8 | Contact with |
| | (2%) | Contact Person |
| (2) Counseling, Checking if | 217 | |
| Really Connected, Pushed | (49%) | |
| Button in Error | | |
| (3) Unplugged from Power | 211 | |
| Source | (48%) | |
| (4) Telephone Set Failure | 7 | |
| | (1%) | |

TABLE 6: MIYAGI PREFECTURE'S ERS RECEPTION SITUATION (2/2)

(Alarm Detected by Sensor)

| | | |
|---|---|---|
| Total Signals Received | 8,940 | |
| Reception Contents | | |
| (1) Abnormality Found | 1 | Death Confirmed |
| | (0%) | |
| (2) No Abnormality Found | 521 | Not Using Own |
| | (6%) | Toilet, etc. |
| (3) Being Away Overnight or in | 7,916 | Report to |
| Hospital with Advance | (88%) | Welfare |
| Notice | | Department |
| | | Made in |
| | | Advance |

## Target Users

Although the target is elderly people living alone throughout the country, anybody living alone can also join. As of February 1990, about 1,000 people are using the service.

## ERS Reception Situation

Up to now, an average of 6 to 8 calls are received each day. Most such calls involve consultations, and are handled by personnel at the reception center who have nursing qualifications. Although true emergency reports constitute a small percentage of the total, the Safety Center handles all contacts by functioning as a "window" for various forms of consultation.

## Contact Persons

Each member needs to register four contact persons (neighbors and relatives).

## Cost Structure

Users are required to bear the following charges:

| | |
|---|---|
| 1. Enrollment Fee | 30,000 ($200) |
| 2. Monthly Membership Fee | 2,800 ($18.70) |
| (ERS user equipment rentalcharge included) | |
| 3. Installation Fee | Actual Expense |
| 4. Call Charges | Actual Expense |

*Items to Be Improved*

1. Striving to establish a management foundation, which is considered to be difficult on a specialized business basis.
2. In consideration of cases in which confirmation of the situation by the Safety Center is not possible, trying to further reinforce the linkage between the private company and local government (ambulance).

## "Hana-Chan" Telephone's ERS

"Hana-Chan" Telephone's ERS was carried out on a trial basis between September 1987 and July 1988, by installing the center at a private retirement home in Tokyo. Target users were 20 elderly people living alone in Tokyo who were seeking human contact.

### Service Features

Besides allowing emergency signals to be sent by only a single touch of the stick control, human-contact service is provided in which the Hana-Chan Telephone center makes phone calls twice a day (morning and afternoon) to ask after users and relays user messages. However, some users have reported they felt the contact service via telephone from the Hana-Chan Telephone Center was somewhat troublesome.

### Development in the Future

Following the trial in Tokyo, the service is now operated in the town of Iwaki in Akita Prefecture, 600km north of Tokyo. A further enrichment of "high-touch services" is planned to provide users with living information, health information, etc., from the center. This will be done by using "off-talk communications," which is NTT's network service that provides information through subscriber lines when they are not in use for telephone calls.

## FUTURE ERS THEMES IN JAPAN

According to a 1987 survey in Tokyo where ERS systems in Japan were carried out at an early stage, ERS has brought about the following direct and indirect effects:

- Actual emergencies of elderly people living alone were dealt with, and help was provided.
- Psychological effects were substantial, as it provided users and their friends and relatives with a sense of comfort and security.
- On an indirect basis, exchanges between users and contact persons developed and mutual understanding was deepened.
- Similarly, users themselves became more active in positive exchanges with people in their communities via the contact persons.

However, Japan's history with ERS is short, and it is presently estimated to cover only 10% of municipalities and serves just 2% of the elderly people throughout the country who are 65 and over and living alone.

One of the most important goals for Japan's elderly welfare policy is to spread and expand ERS to older people living alone throughout the country as the society continues its rapid aging. Moreover, the next goal is to expand the service to households consisting of frail elderly people, and frail elderly who are alone during the daytime (nighttime). To achieve these goals, the following matters have been pointed out by those concerned:

### Cost-Bearing Measures

For example, in the case of adding 100 more ERS users, the cost of the user equipment alone will be about 10 million ($66,667). Accompanying the increase of users, moreover, is the need to install additional ERS center equipment and provide for an increase in personnel. For this reason, and in terms of administrative service as well, it is necessary to further promote measures for efficient ERS operation, such as the introduction of recipient cost-bearing, and entrusting ERS to the private sector.

### Establishing the Environment to Spread ERS

- Attempting to standardize system configuration and operation methods in order to provide for an easier selection and a sense of safety in using private ERS.

- Attempting to organize related businesses in order to raise the level of ERS.

### Improvement of Services

It is necessary to improve ERS services in the future. The improved service could include the "human contact service" which, like "HANA-CHAN" telephone, offers consultation to help members meet the needs of daily life and provides information on living, health, etc., and escort service to the hospital in cases of non-emergency on receipt of user request, which can be provided by private rescue service companies.

### Integration with Social Systems, Such as Emergency Medical Services, Fire-Defense and Crime-Prevention Services

- To carry out prompt life-saving activities, attempting to organically link ERS with existing systems, such as the emergency medical information service and Dial 119 (fire and ambulance).
- In carrying forward the integration with social services, it is necessary to review the existing ways of sharing between administrative and private services.

### Reduction of Burden on Contact Persons Who Play an Important Role in ERS, and Securing Personnel

- Focusing its eyes on this problem, a taxi company has started providing service to confirm the situation when users send emergency signals by dispatching taxi drivers rather than contact persons to visit a user's home.

### Improvement of System

- Resolving trade-offs such as making the push buttons on emergency transmitters (such as the pendant type) less prone to being triggered accidentally, while still making them easy to operate when real emergencies are encountered.
- Realizing systems that will automatically send signals by detecting physiological abnormalities, etc., in case of emergencies where the user cannot even push the button.

- Establishing methods whereby sensor warnings of abnormal situations, are reported without a long time lapse.
- Modifying the current system that covers users at home to one that can cope with emergencies when they are away from home as well.

## REFERENCES

1. Elderly Service Providers Association, "Present Situation of Emergency Response Services," May 1989.

2. Geriatric Welfare Development Center, "Guide to Geriatric Welfare," September 1989.

3. City of Tokyo, "Evaluation of Emergency Response Systems (Report)," November 1986.

4. Tokyo Retirement Home, "Report on R&D of Emergency Response Systems for Elderly People Living Alone," March 1986.

# THE NETHERLANDS

# Organizing and Financing PRS by a Health Insurance Fund

## Jan Bok

There are two separate sources of financing health care in the Netherlands. The first is the compulsory health care system for workers below a certain income level. This covers 60% of the population. Above that income level, you must be privately insured.

Fifteen years ago Silver Cross, the largest not-for-profit private health insurance fund in the Netherlands, extended its geographic area of health-risk coverage to include the entire world. At present, there is a 100% standard coverage of health care costs around the globe, wherever the insured person is inclined to go. Extending the area of coverage, however, required the establishment of an international emergency centre so that insured members in need of immediate assistance could be helped with language, financial and primarily medical problems all over the world, whether as a result of an accident or of health complications. Very special cost-containment measures were built in.

Silver Cross' Emergency Response Organization for members abroad, named EuroCross, serves more than 16 million members at present–five million Dutch, six million Belgian, two million British, and a considerable number Canadian, Israeli and African. The EuroCross emergency centre is operational 24 hours a day, every day of the year. The crew that operates

Jan Bok is affiliated with Eurocross Alarm Centre.

*101*

the centre is able to give assistance in almost any language. They depend upon medical advice from doctors.

Silver Cross, in its capacity as a health insurer, is increasingly being confronted with overconsumption of health care facilities since market supply by far exceeds demands. There is an overuse of hospital beds and specialist care and a shortage of nursing homes. People stayed in the hospital longer than medically necessary.

Personal response services for frail persons have been established for a number of reasons: To reduce substantially the costs to be met by Silver Cross Health insurance; and to be able to optimize services rendered to the policy holders.

Twenty-four hour stand-by emergency assistance is provided by the PRS Center called "Actionline." It is called Actionline, not Lifeline, because it implies not only life questions, but also questions of safety. The term Actionline is registered.

The Actionline emergency center operates all over the Netherlands, not only on behalf of the affiliated members of Silver Cross, but also for cooperating sick funds and several small municipalities which cannot afford to monitor PRS. We subsidize those small organizations.

The center receives signals of members in possession of PRS equipment exclusively. The center offers immediate emergency relief actions in the event of medical emergencies and matters of risk and/or danger in and around the house. The philosophy of the ERS center is that people want to talk to people. Therefore we have no automatic answering equipment. We also believe that people do not want to be out of touch for long periods.

Our equipment includes a portable wireless trigger with a push button and also a pull switch. It is highly reliable, with a high frequency signal. Our system insures privacy and the certainty that it works. There is vocal contact within one minute of the signal, with a two way voice system. There is a self-testing procedure, and emergency power. At the monitoring center there is immediate identification of the caller, and recording with a printed record of calls.

PRS enables affiliated members to remain longer within their familiar surroundings without depending on health care schemes. This is an absolute necessity since contrary to the general tendency of increasing demographic figures of aged citizens, general public facilities on behalf of the aged and disabled are progressively decreasing in number.

Silver Cross Health Insurance distributes home monitors on a loan basis to:

* Patients recently discharged from the hospital but in need of constant monitoring.

- Patients in a terminal health condition.
- Elderly citizens in need of constant availability of home care.

Furthermore, Silver Cross sells monitors to insured members who appreciate PRS membership for safety reasons. Most of them are women.

This has also proved to be a welcome solution to many people in view of the present rapid increase in criminal activities. At the same time, PRS has made reduction of the costs of health care feasible.

The combination of health insurer and a personal response center is, from a management point of view, efficient and effective. Organizing PRS can stimulate substitution of home care for expensive in-patient care, in the interest of the insured as well as the insurer.

Insured persons buying the PRS system obtain an instrument to make them independent from health facilities as long as they would rather stay in their own surroundings.

Silver Cross members do not pay anything as long as the equipment is loaned. The ones who bought the system (approximately $700 U.S.) pay for the connection to the PRS center at approximately $8 (U.S.) per month.

We find emergency response systems to be effective in meeting our management goals, promoting home care to avoid expensive inpatient care. Our costs are low because we can use the existing Eurocross Emergency Response Center. Selling the concept of ERS to the private market is difficult. People do not want ERS just because of advanced age. Even at 85 they say they are not "old enough." It would help to make a trigger with universal functions which would be more easily accepted.

In closing, I must point out that the problem of financing health care is an international one. I propose that we continue to share our ideas, to make available to all, commercial or not for profit, the best technology, and to insist on the highest quality.

# From Alarm Systems
# to Smart Houses

Frank J. M. Vlaskamp

SUMMARY. The percentage of senior citizens in the Netherlands will rise in coming years. The expected percentage for the year 2010 of persons over age 65 in the total population is 15%. More persons over age 65 than ever before will continue to live in their own environment. Emergency response systems (ERS) can support independent living. The most common type of organization distributing ERS is a small, partly subsidized local alarm organization run by a social welfare office for the elderly. Government subsidy has been reduced in recent years which has motivated small organizations to join together into larger regional organizations in order to get a more solid financial base. On the other hand new semi-commercial and commercial organizations have come into being. These developments are part of the growing importance of home care, leading to more medical applications of ERS.

User satisfaction with ERS is high. Portable triggers can enhance the effectiveness of the system. However, many users do not wear the portable trigger when feeling well. Future technical developments will result in multifunctionality of ERS-devices. In the long term the hardware of today will be integrated in a multimedia home terminal replacing the telephone. The portable trigger will remain the only specific hardware at home for ERS.

## DEMOGRAPHIC INFORMATION

In most countries of the EEC population growth is decreasing. In some countries even the absolute size of the population will be smaller in the year 2010 than it is now.

---

Frank J. M. Vlaskamp is affiliated with the Institute for Rehabilitation Research, The Netherlands.

*105*

This development is caused by a sharp drop in the birth rates and a longer life expectancy. Both developments result in an increasing percentage of persons over age 65.

In the Netherlands this percentage will increase from 12% in 1985 to 15% in 2010. Not very high when compared with W. Germany (21% in 2010) (see Table 1).

A high percentage of elderly means that a large part of the population is not vocationally active. It also means that a greater part of the labor force

Table 1 -   Population size, population growth, and percentage persons over age 65 in Europe, in 1960, 1985 and 2010

| | Pop. (*mill.) | | | Growth (%) | | % of persons over age 65 | | |
|---|---|---|---|---|---|---|---|---|
| | 1960 | 1985 | 2010 | 1960-85 | 1985-2010 | 1960 | 1985 | 2010 |
| Belgium | 9.1 | 9.9 | 9.4 | + 9% | - 5% | 12% | 14% | 17% |
| W.Germany | 55.1 | 61.1 | 57.8 | +11% | - 5% | 11% | 15% | 21% |
| Denmark | 4.6 | 5.1 | 5.0 | +11% | - 2% | 11% | 15% | 17% |
| France | 45.5 | 55.1 | 58.8 | +21% | + 7% | 12% | 13% | 16% |
| Greece | 8.3 | 9.9 | 10.6 | +19% | + 7% | 8% | 13% | 17% |
| Ireland | 2.8 | 3.5 | 4.8 | +25% | +37% | 11% | 11% | 9% |
| Italy | 50.0 | 57.1 | 55.7 | +14% | - 3% | 9% | 13% | 18% |
| Luxembourg | 0.3 | 0.4 | 0.4 | +17% | + 1% | 11% | 13% | 15% |
| NETHERLANDS | 11.4 | 14.5 | 15.8 | +27% | + 9% | 9% | 12% | 15% |
| Portugal | 9.0 | 10.1 | 11.7 | +12% | +16% | 8% | 12% | 12% |
| Spain | 30.3 | 38.4 | 41.2 | +27% | + 7% | 8% | 12% | 15% |
| United Kingdom | 52.2 | 56.5 | 59.4 | + 8% | + 5% | 12% | 15% | 16% |

Source:   van der Wijst, C.A., De demografie van de twaalf in cijfers, in SER-bulletin, Juni 1989, p. 9-10.

and national income will be needed for home care and institutional care for the elderly. On the other hand, lower birth rates reduce the number of youths to be educated, and increase the participation of women in the labor market. Furthermore the coming generation of elderly will be more socially active, healthy and self-supporting than former generations.

In Dutch society there is a tendency to integrate younger age categories (55-65 years) into the definition of "the elderly." A new "senior" is being defined who is socially active, healthy, financially independent, and knowing how to stand up for his rights. This positive image is propagated by the associations of the elderly, life insurance companies and pension funds, real estate companies, travel agencies, etc. "Service" is the keyword instead of "Care," when speaking of provisions for the new seniors. Dutch government policy is aimed at a reduction of the percentage of elderly living in medical and non-medical settings (now about 11% of those age 65+). Living independently in their own environment can be economically profitable and is preferred by many seniors for psychological and social reasons.

Emergency response systems are considered to be one of the means to support independent living (see Photo).

## NUMBER OF PERSONS USING ERS

In the Netherlands there is no central registration of persons using ERS. The consequence is that no national statistics on ERS exist. The only way to discover the facts about ERS is to start an investigation among about 250 organizations distributing ERS, importers and manufacturers of equipment. In 1986 the Institute for Rehabilitation Research conducted such an investigation. In 1986 the estimated number of persons using ERS was about 15000 elderly (about 1% of the age group 65+) and 1500 younger handicapped persons. Since 1986 the number of persons using ERS was quickly rising. In areas where ERS had been available for some years the average percentage was about 3% of the age group 65 years and older. It was assumed that after the introduction of ERS a saturation point would gradually be reached, being about 3% of the age group. The saturation point would be reached with 50000 users in The Netherlands. Using a lot of fragmentary information as a basis for a tentative guess the number of persons using ERS can now be estimated at 30000 (1990)(see Tables 2 and 3).

PHOTO: The leading product on the Dutch market ESTAFETTE features two-way speech, programmable telephone numbers, and a spoken alarm message.

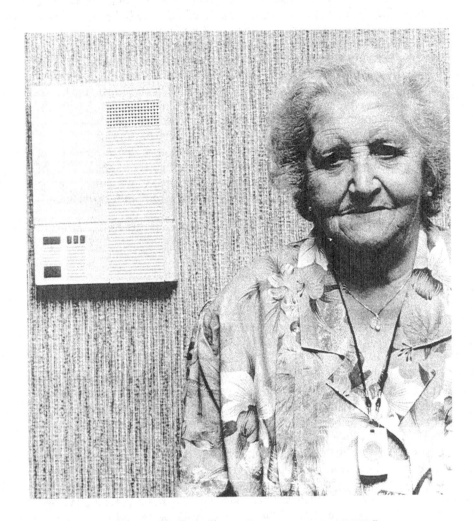

## CHARACTERISTICS OF THOSE USING ERS

Impairments come with age. Many elderly have impairments, especially in mobility, endurance, eating hard food, hearing and vision. Most people continue independent living, even when impairments develop. This

Table 2 - Number of persons using Emergency Response Services

(ERS) for frail persons living alone

number of persons over age 65          = 1.6 million

number of elderly using ERS (1986)     = 15000

number of young handicapped using ERS (1986)    = 1500

------------------------------------------------------------------

---Source:   Vlaskamp, F.J.M., Alarmeringssystemen voor ouderen en

gehandicapten, Instituut voor Revalidatie Vraagstukken, Hoensbroek,

1988, p. 20-21.

------------------------------------------------------------------

will be possible when provisions are made to adapt the house, when additional care is available, when the social, cultural and physical home environment encourages staying independent.

The Institute for Rehabilitation Research has conducted a nationwide research among people using ERS. Some results are presented in Tables 4 and 5.

Many people using ERS need help with daily life activities, such as shopping, cooking, kneeling, and climbing stairs (Table 4). Among people using ERS the percentage of younger handicapped is low (about 6%). The majority of ERS users is of the female sex (78%). Most ERS-users are living alone (84%). Their own judgement of their health situation is relatively favorable. In only a few cases ERS is used by bedridden patients. About 30% of ERS-users have problems with hearing and vision.

## TECHNOLOGY, STRUCTURE AND ECONOMICS

### Most Common Types of Organization

In Table 6 the most common types of organization in the Netherlands are given. The points of difference are the place where the alarm message is first received (control center or volunteer aid) and the person giving help (volunteer aid or professional). Family members, neighbors, friends, have always played an important role in ERS as volunteer aid. In some small

**Table 3 - Estimation of development of the use of Emergency Response Services (ERS) for frail persons living alone**

Percentage of persons over age 65 with ERS (1986)     +/- 1%

Percentage of persons over age 65 with ERS in

communities where alarm organizations are

operational for a number of years (= estimated

saturation point, based on experience)     +/- 3%


Number of elderly using ERS when saturation

point is reached     +/- 50.000


Estimated number of elderly using ERS (1990)     +/- 30.000

----------------------------------------------------------------


Source: Vermijs, P., and Wijnen-Sponselee, M.Th., Basisrapport Sociale Alarmering als ondersteuning van be thuiszorg, GIMD/PSSA, Tilburg, 1988, p. 12-19. Vlaskamp, F.J.M., Alarmeringssystemen voor ouderen en gehandicapten, Instituut voor Revalidatie Vraagstukken, Hoenbroke, 1988, p. 20-21.

----------------------------------------------------------------


organizations without a special control center pre-recorded alarm messages are sent first to volunteer aids. When these persons do not react the message is sent to a 24 hour a day manned control center of a police department, a fire station or a hospital.

In most organizations the control center comes first. It can be expected that this will be the standard way to organize ERS in the future.

Smaller organizations will gradually be incorporated in large cooperatives with specialized control centers.

Having a control center gives the opportunity to take advantage of an

<u>Table 4 - Characteristics of those using Emergency Response</u>

<u>Services (ERS) for frail persons living alone</u>

|  | Can you perform these activities without help? |
|---|---|
| Activities | Not possible to do<br>on my own, in % of cases<br>(100% =239 cases) |
| walking up/down the stairs | 34% |
| going outdoors | 16% |
| going to the toilet | 2% |
| washing face/hands | 2% |
| bath/shower/washing body | 4% |
| getting dressed | 2% |
| going in/out of bed | 2% |
| kneeling/bending | 35% |
| combing hair | 2% |
| go out shopping | 44% |
| cooking dinner | 34% |

------------------------------------------------------------------

Source: Vlaskamp, F.J.M., Alarmeringssystemen voor
ouderen en gehandicapten, Instituut voor
Revalidatie Vraagstukken, Hoensbroek, 1988, p.
68

------------------------------------------------------------------

important technological development of ERS: the speech link. The speech
link makes it possible to differentiate between alarm messages: between
false alarms and real alarms, whether medical urgency exists, etc. When
the speech link was introduced there was some opposition against it ("Big

Table 5 -      Characteristics of those using
               Emergency Response Services (ERS)
               for frail persons living alone, age,
               sex, living conditions, hearing and
               vision.

- Age          (100% = 239 cases)

< 60 years         6%

61-70 years       12%

71-80 years       42%

81-90 years       36%

91-100 years       3%

- Sex

male              22%

female            78%

- Living conditions

living alone      84%

with other(s)     16%

- State of health (own judgement)

very good          8%

good              36%

fair              41%

bad               13%

very bad           2%

- Confined to bed for long periods

permanent          2%

> 4 weeks a year            5%

TABLE 5 (continued)

```
< 4 weeks a year        2%

not confined to bed     91%

- Hearing problems (conversation)

yes         27%

no          73%

- Vision problems (reading papers)

yes         34%

no          66%
```

---

Source:  Vlaskamp, F.J.M., Alarmeringssystemen voor

ouderen en gehandicapten, Instituut voor

Revalidatie Vraagstukken, Hoensbroek, 1988,

pp. 66-67.

---

brother talking and listening"). At this moment speech links are nearly a standard provision in new devices.

The availability of a speech link also makes a flexible choice between professional and volunteer aid possible, depending on the situation. Very few organizations have only professional aids.

Three types of organizations can be distinguished. First organizations subsidized by government funds and run by organizations working for the elderly. Second, semi-commercial organizations run by home care services. And third, commercial alarm organizations.

## The Subsidized Sector (Most Common Type of Organization)

The most common type of organization distributing ERS is a small, partly subsidized, local alarm organization run by a social welfare organization for the elderly. Most organizations have less than 50 subscribers.

Table 6 - Most common types of organization

| User | Who receives message? | Who gives help? |
|------|----------------------|-----------------|
| user | 24 hours a day control centre | volunteer aid professional when needed |
| user | volunteer aid | volunteer aid professional when needed |
| | back up when volunteers do not react: 24 hours a day control centre | professional aid |
| user | 24 hours a day manned control centre | volunteer aid and professional, depends on user and situation |
| user | 24 hours a day control centre | professional aid |

Acceptance of new subscribers is restricted, using criteria as: age, living alone, psychological conditions like feeling unsafe, and lonely, social conditions, emergency situations in the past, or being on the waiting list of a home for the elderly. The assessment of applications for an alarm system is done by a so-called "indication committee."

Subscription rates are low (about 7 US-dollars a month) and paid by the monitored person. Since 1984 the Dutch government has promoted independent living for the elderly. One of the goals was a reduction of the percentage of elderly living in institutions (from 9% to 7%). At the same time the quality of home care, housing, distribution of meals, services of homes for the elderly for non-residents was improved. Emergency alarm services were considered as one of the means to support independent living. The Dutch government funded the investments necessary to create local alarm organizations.

The government subsidy flow for investments declined recently. The responsibility for implementation of government policy concerning the elderly was partly transferred to communities. The subsidies in the beginning years made the creation possible of small organizations with no sound financial basis. The decline of subsidies threatens the continuity of these organizations. As a consequence there is a tendency to join organizations into regional organizations, retaining help in case of emergency at a local level.

## The Semi-Commercial Sector (New on the Market)

Home care services are developing a full 24 hours a day, 7 days a week telephone service. Home care (nursing, home help) will be more client oriented in the future, and will not restrict its activities to ordinary office hours. Communication centers are established, staffed with qualified nurses. These centers mediate between questions and calls for help coming from people at home and (after screening) professional workers or volunteer aids. The working area is a region or province. The provision of emergency alarm service matches well with the goals of home care services. The growing importance of home care technology increases the demand for telemonitoring of patients and medical devices. Home care services are better equipped for these tasks than the traditional alarm organizations for the elderly. Furthermore the activities of home care organizations are not limited to the elderly.

Some home care services have established new semi-commercial organizations for the operation of their alarm services. These non-subsidized organizations usually have no restricted acceptance of subscribers. Lack of subsidy has some advantage for new subscribers: they do not have to meet the criteria of an "indication committee," evaluating each new case. The subscription rate is about 12 US dollars monthly, paid by the monitored person.

### The Commercial Sector

The commercial sector has always been active in the market of alarm services. The manufacturers and importers of the hardware, of course, address themselves to all profit and non-profit alarm organizations. Speaking of personal emergency alarm services, a few organizations are providing services on a for profit basis. Commercial organizations have an unlimited working area (mostly nationwide). Personal emergency alarm service is only one alarm activity of these organizations, other activities include intruder alarm, fire alarm and industrial alarm. The number of subscribers of each organization is high when compared with the non-profit sector. The subscription rates are about $20-30 US monthly, paid by the monitored person. Commercial organizations have no selection criteria for acceptance of clients.

The market share of the (few) profit organizations is relatively small, due to the large subsidies of the Dutch government for non-profit organizations working for the elderly. However there is some overlap between the profit and non-profit sector. Some non-profit organizations have their alarm calls processed by a nationwide commercial alarm service. The Joint Medical Service (G.M.D.), the national social security administration for people under 65 years of age, prefers to make contracts with a commercial or semi-commercial ERS organization with a large working area, instead of making arrangements with a great number of local organizations. For handicapped persons under 65 years of age, alarm systems can be obtained as a provision paid for by social security.

Some commercial organizations are decentralizing their national control centers and forming a few regional centers. There are practical reasons to do this. A regional control center can gather much information about the "social map" of the area. Using the speech link a better communication with dialect speaking inhabitants is possible. Distribution lines for equipment are shorter for a regional control center. Decentralization is made more economic by the increasing number of people using ERS and by technical developments in equipment, giving the opportunity to connect different brands of equipment to one center. It can be expected that the regional center will be the level of organization of ERS in the future. Small non-profit organizations will gradually join regional centers for the processing of alarm calls.

## OPERATIONS

### Equipment

During the last decade more than twenty manufacturers and importers of alarm equipment were active on the Dutch market. In the beginning there was a coming and going of small manufacturers and importers. In a study of the Joint Medical Service (GMD, 1987) manufacturers and importers were invited to send in equipment for evaluation of technical quality. Only twelve brands could meet the minimal technical requirements formulated by the GMD. These twelve brands were evaluated. The most frequent critical remarks were:

portable trigger
1. force to operate switch too high
2. no battery check
3. limited working distance
4. not water-proof

home unit
1. not enough capacity of back-up battery
2. difficult to reset
3. no alarm button on home unit
4. no message when back-up battery is functioning

Quality research by a well-respected institution like the Joint Medical Service can set standards, which can be taken into account by industry.

The market-leading products of today have many features in common, such as:

1. speech link
2. portable trigger
3. alarms are processed by a control center
4. battery check on portable trigger
5. possibility to connect other alarm switches
6. battery back-up for home unit

### Alarm Instructions for the Monitored Person

The instructions for the user describing in which cases the alarm should be used are an important issue. Too strict rules can be a barrier to use the alarm in emergency cases. No restriction can result in demotivation of helpers when their assistance is asked in cases in which the monitored person could solve the situation on his own.

The problem is that each monitored person has his own interpretation of the rules and of the situation. The most followed policy of alarm organizations is to encourage triggering an alarm when the monitored person thinks something is wrong, and to correct on the individual level when someone uses the alarm unnecessarily. The speech link, a standard-option of equipment now on the market, makes immediate evaluation of alarm calls possible. This reduces the problem of unnecessary alarm calls.

### User Resistance

User resistance against personal alarm systems is low. People apply for an alarm system, so there is self-selection of people who have a favorable attitude. Some housing projects for the elderly have alarm systems as a standard provision. People who move into such a project take its availability as a matter of course. However, when alarms are to be effective there is some discipline required from the monitored person. Many people resist wearing a portable trigger all day. In a number of potentially dangerous situations the portable trigger is not within reach (in the bathroom, in the kitchen). At least one third of the monitored persons do not wear the portable trigger when feeling well. Freedom of choice for the individual as to when to wear the portable trigger means some reduction in the effectiveness of the emergency response system.

## User Satisfaction

User satisfaction with the alarm system is high. The availability of a portable trigger contributes to user satisfaction. However, some critical remarks concerning the portable trigger are to be made; inadvertent operation of the switch is possible, a portable trigger is an ugly thing to wear, irritation of the neck may be caused by the cord.

People who have experienced a real alarm situation are, generally speaking, satisfied with the way help was organized. Our research showed that no 100% effective help was obtained. This was caused by faulty equipment, mistakes of the user and the control center personnel, and slow or inadequate help. A total failure of the system was reported in 3 of 65 emergency cases.

## Frequency of Emergencies

Frequencies of emergencies show much variation between organizations. The reported frequencies are a consequence of:

- definition of what is considered as an emergency
- record keeping
- purposes a monitored person is allowed to use the alarm for
- selection of user groups (no selection, medical cases only, or social, psychological and medical cases)

Our research showed that emergencies do not occur frequently. The average frequency was not higher than once a year. There is much difference on the individual level. Many subscribers never cause an alarm, few subscribers are frequent users.

## Integration with Medical and Social Services

Personal emergency response devices are part of a group of provisions aimed at the support of independent living (home care technology). Home care technology is a new branch of medical technology. Home care itself can be defined as:

The entire system of care, nursing, treatment, counselling of clients living at home, that performs its task using self-care, care by persons in the direct social environment, volunteer aid and/or additional professional care, and is aimed at support of the client to maintain himself living at home. (National Council for Public Health, the Netherlands)

Integration of Personal Emergency Response Systems with medical and social services in the Netherlands is far from complete. In fact the Dutch home care system is not a unity. Home care is financed by the Dutch National Health Service, private medical insurance companies, social security, government funds and contributions of patients.

The services are delivered by a number of professionals, such as the general practitioner, the district nurse, the home help, and distribution of meals. There is a lack of coordination between institutional care and home care. Until now the organization of home care has been determined more by the different goals of each organization delivering services than by needs of the individual patient. In recent years the necessity of more integration of the home care system was advocated. An important matter in this discussion is the possibility for those who need help to address themselves to only one organization for intake and assessment. This organization is also responsible for a "care-program," tuned to the individual needs, in which the contributions of the different home care disciplines are indicated. This kind of integration of home care is still in an experimental stage.

Most personal emergency systems are run by local social welfare organizations for the elderly. These organizations can give an adequate response to emergencies, because of their knowledge of the local home care organizations. Their target group consists of those elderly that are at risk but do not require constant medical attention. Welfare organizations for the elderly are less qualified for the monitoring of (bedridden) patients and medical equipment. Monitoring of patients requires specific medical knowledge and responsibility. Home care organizations have more affinity with patients requiring medical attention. Alarm organizations are being developed by home care organizations. In the long run these organizations can be a strong competitor on the alarm market, because they can accept both medical cases and people who want an alarm system only for safety reasons.

Home care has also become an issue for medical insurance organizations. With adequate home care, hospital stay can be shortened or prevented. An active policy concerning home care shows to be a success, contributing to the quality of care, well being of patients, and reduction of medical expenses. Several medical insurance organizations are developing national networks for home care. Emergency response systems are utilized to facilitate contact with professional nurses. Medical insurance organizations are also developing personal response services for people who want an alarm for safety. In some policies the option of getting an alarm is given, in order to support independent living.

## BENEFITS OF EMERGENCY RESPONSE SYSTEMS

The benefits of emergency response systems can be described on the individual level and on the social level. Emergency response systems are a relatively cheap but effective provision used to support independent living.

### Medical or Psychological Benefits

There are two aspects to the benefit of an emergency response system for the individual. Firstly, it gives a feeling of safety, which can be enjoyed every day when no emergencies occur. Secondly, it makes the organization of adequate help possible in the usually rare moments of emergency.

Without ERS the monitoring task is done by family members or people in the direct neighborhood. A number of evaluation studies showed that the frequency of visits did not decrease when an alarm system was installed. People who pay visits feel themselves freed from the monitoring task, their visit is now more clearly considered as a social call.

For medical cases emergency response systems can help the nursing of patients at home. Alarm calls can be used to request medical service and not only in case of emergency.

### Cost Savings and Cost Avoidance

Emergency response systems are part of a number of provisions and services aimed at continuation of independent living. The cost of institutionalization is high: about $1600 US dollars monthly for a single person in a home for the elderly. Living independently does not imply that these costs can be totally avoided. Costs of daily living, domestic assistance, provisions at home, and the monthly rent have to be met. The balance of cost savings and cost avoidance has to be made on the individual level. When permanent intensive home care is needed, professional help at home will be less efficient than hospitalization. For instance, twelve hours a week home help already costs about $900 US dollars a month. On the other hand many people can stay independent when minor provisions and assistance are available. An emergency response system is one of the means for support of independent living, but seldom is the availability of an alarm system alone the criterion that determines whether to go or not to go to a home for the elderly. Calculation of the cost/savings balance of the use of emergency response systems is not very useful. In fact an emergency response system turns out to be a cheap provision, when compared with the cost of many other provisions and professional help.

## EXPECTED FUTURE TECHNICAL DEVELOPMENTS

Will the technical development of personal emergency response systems come to an end? For the most frequent application of today, the possibility of causing an alarm when in distress, these devices have reached maturity.

Many features once were an option of some products. Now they are built-in standard features of the leading products on the market.

Such as:
- portable trigger
- speech-link
- battery back-up of home unit
- power failure signals of home unit and trigger
- automatic alert of center in case of power failure

All those features can be expected to be available in a good home unit. But what can technical developments add to the performance of today's home unit? Not much, if alarm units should stay devices dedicated to one function. However, there are some developments towards a multifunctional system. In this multifunctional system two kinds of integration take place. First there is a tendency to integrate more alarm-functions in the system (such as smoke alarm, sensors of the water supply, low room temperature alarm, possibility of connecting medical devices).

In the second place there is a tendency to integrate non-alarm functions in the system (such as auto-dial functions for normal telephone calls, loud-speaking telephone, possibility of pick up the telephone using the portable trigger). There are arguments for and against these developments. One-function alarm systems can be easily installed and removed. Sensors can make the installation more complex. When more types of alarm are possible, coding or artificial speech messages are necessary. The control center must know what type of alarm is given. There should be strict procedures for each type of alarm. Otherwise there is a chance of an inadequate response to the call. Adding non-alarm functions to the units can disguise the most vital function of the unit: sending out an alarm call.

It can be expected that in the long term the portable trigger will communicate with a standard home terminal which will be introduced by the telephone companies as a replacement for the telephone. These terminals will be able to send and receive speech, video and data (so-called Integrated Broadband Communication Terminals, IBC). The portable trigger will finally remain the only hardware at home for personal emergency response systems.

## REFERENCES

Fontein, P., Thuiszorg, een zorg, in: Health Lines, International Health Development Foundation, Newsletter Vol 3/3 April 1990.

Gemeenschappelijke Medische Dienst (GMD), Warenonderzoek alarmeringsapparatuur, Amsterdam, 1987.

Gemeenschappelijke Medische Dienst (GMD), Beoordelingscriteria '89, Amsterdam 1989.

Institute for Rehabilitation Research (IRV), Research Report 1988, Hoensbroek, 1989, p. 103-107.

Research Institute for Consumer Affairs (RICA), Dispersed Alarms; a guide for organizations installing systems, London, 1986.

SIGO, Projectplan Intelligente Woningen voor Gehandicapten en Ouderen, Hoensbroek, 1989.

Vermijs, P., and Wijnen-Sponselee, M.Th., Basisrapport Sociale Alarmering als ondersteuning van de thuiszorg, GIMD/PSSA, Tilburg, 1988, p. 12-19.

Vlaskamp, F.J.M., Alarmering als aanvulling op de voorzieningen voor thuiszorg, in: Smeets, J.W. (ed.), Thuiszorg en Techniek, Delft, 1988, p. 103-110.

Vlaskamp, F.J.M., en Beks, M.C.M., Alarmeringssystemen voor ouderen en gehandicapten, Institute for Rehabilitation Research, Hoensbroek, 1988.

Wiersema, M.I., Een toekomst voor thuiszorg?, in: Health Lines, International Health Development Foundation, Newsletter Vol 3/3 april 1990.

van der Wijst, C.A., De demografie van de twaalf in cijfers, in: SER-bulletin, juni 1989, p. 9-10.

# NEW ZEALAND

# Mid-Range Technology:
# A New Zealand Perspective

## W. Randolph Herman

New Zealand is a small nation of topographically diverse islands surrounded and divided by water; it is situated in the South Pacific Basin, 1500 miles East of Australia. Despite its relative geographic isolation, rapid social and economic changes have occurred during the last ten years. This is evidenced by limiting government ownership, decentralizing and regionalizing control, moving toward bi-cultural development, and competing actively in the international marketplace. The current reliance on a market-led economy has had a major impact on product development and service delivery, especially in the area of human services. This paper will examine the Emergency Response System (ERS) in the New Zealand context. ERS is an example of mid-range technology that can assist the elderly and disabled in their work, leisure, and activities of daily living, as well as provide a low cost way to assist people to safely remain in their own homes. Although numerous communities throughout the country have ERS, little research has been done, specifically in this area.

## DEMOGRAPHY

People are living longer and needs are changing. The heterogeneous nature of New Zealand society has more recently been acknowledged and

W. Randolph Herman resides in Maitland, FL.

its complex social context requires a reassessment of perceptions of the stages of life and what human effectiveness really is. When human capacities diminish, caring for people should be based on a realistic understanding of their needs and a moral obligation to make full use of their potential.

There are currently 3.3 million people in New Zealand and there has been a dramatic shift in the age cohorts of that population. In 1961 children under the age of 5 and adults over the age of 60 both equalled 12% of the total population. By 1985 adults over 60 had doubled, equalling 482,000 or 14.6% of the population. This trend toward an aging population is occurring not only in New Zealand but all around the world. Added to this potentially large population who will have a variety of needs in relationship to their aging, is the imbalance of the distribution of population in New Zealand as a whole. In 1986, 73.8% of the population was in the North Island, with only 26.2% in the South Island.

To demonstrate cost benchmarks for what the country is facing now and will be facing in the future, the following provides some indication. Loans for home alterations in 1986 made to the Department of Social Welfare equalled $2,192,000. Respite care for disabled children and adults equalled $3,316,000. Supporting loans for motor vehicle adaptation were $587,000 on 134 cars, and funding for disability aids, such as walking frames and prosthetic appliances, was $718,000.

Under the Social Security Act of 1964 Part 2, the Health Department is responsible for dealing with a variety of areas for the elderly and disabled. This includes the free supply of artificial orthopedic appliances, crutches, manual wheelchairs, colostomy appliances, subsidizing breast prostheses, and wigs. The supplementary benefit paid by the Department of Health for artificial aids went from $168,000 in 1981 to $444,000 in 1986. This large increase will be insignificant to the increase society is facing as the demography continues to change. Department of Health payments for old people's homes and hospital building subsidies for 1986 was $5,243,153. They are active in supporting religious and welfare organizations who provide over 18,628 home and hospital beds for the elderly as well as hospital boards and area health boards that maintain 907 old people's homes beds and 2,880 home beds for the elderly. The budget for the New Zealand Disabilities Resource Centre was $968,000 in 1986-87 and will be over a million dollars in 1988 (Palmerston North Hospital Board Financial Estimates and Annual Statistical Report, year ending March 1987).

The Accident Compensation Act of 1972 which took effect in April 1974 ensures that New Zealanders are provided with safety promotion, prompt and effective rehabilitation services, and prompt and reasonable compensation for accidents. Again, the statistics show certain populations being highlighted at risk and in need of care and technological devices to ensure that their life-style can be maintained. During 1985 the largest category of accidents was accidental falls. The people who had these falls also had the longest aggregate stay in hospital. A majority of them were fractures of femurs and fell within the 60+ population–in total 114,806 hospital days. The fourth largest category of accidents was motor vehicles and they compile the second largest aggregate number of days in hospital.

Department of Social Welfare, Department of Health and Accident Compensation statistics certainly contribute to the overall picture of current need and potential need as the population in New Zealand undergoes a rapid age distribution change. There will be progressively fewer young people, more people in working groups and much more in the elderly age groups. Those aged 60 years and over will increase from 14.9% to 22.5% of the population.

The statistics on disabilities are more difficult in that disabilities range from short-term to permanent and not all people are forthcoming in defining themselves as disabled. Particularly in the case of the elderly, there is the added complication of multiple disabilities so that getting an accurate measure of the level of disability in New Zealand is difficult. It is estimated that close to 400,000 people in New Zealand have some form of disability which requires attention, either medical or social service in nature. Future planning and future service delivery must "come to grips" with a complex set of variables. Service delivery is further complicated by the population distribution, not only in the North and South Island, but between main urban areas, secondary minor urban areas and rural areas. Sixty-seven point five percent of the population live in main urban areas in New Zealand, 16% live in secondary minor urban areas, and 16.2% in rural areas. The urban drift and the major drift to the North Island is having a significant impact on allocation of resources and development of services.

## POLITICAL AND SOCIAL FACTORS

Researching technology and disabilities and aging in a world filled with absurdities is a paradox in itself. In Northern Ireland, for example, in the last 20 years the war has caused over 30,000 casualties. In the next state–the Republic of Ireland–a firm makes a profit by producing prosthetic knees for those people who lost them in the war. In England, a group of scientists and engineers over 70 years of age has banded together to form an emergency team to assess and clean up after nuclear accidents. They offer their expertise and their limited life-span so that younger people can be spared the lethal effects of radiation. In the USA, where by the year 2030, 21.5% of the population will be over 65 and one state governor commented that "the elderly have a duty to die and get out of the way," a move is currently under way to promote the refusal of life-extending medical services for those over 75 years of age. Less dramatic absurdities in New Zealand include new public buildings which defy current building codes and are without wheelchair access, wards for elderly without technology to give them access to toileting in the most dignified manner, and the profoundly deaf are unable to call any hospital when the technology for doing so is reasonably priced and available. In a technocratic society dominated by the able-bodied, the elderly and disabled have minimal currency, despite demographic statistics and social indicators that plainly paint a different picture.

New Zealand, like many other western nations, is beginning to address these discrepancies. The Report of the Royal Commission on Social Policy provides a comprehensive overview of the needs of the elderly and disabled (Koopman-Boyden, 1988; Hunt, 1988). The current lack of a comprehensive national policy on aging and the elderly is reflected in the wide variation in availability and quality of in-home and institutional care. By the year 2011, there will be a 40% growth in the number of 65 to 79-year-olds and a 121.7% increase in those over 80. In the Maori population there will be a 300% increase in those over the age of 65.

To promote health and to maximize independency, the provision of adequate social services, income support and access to appropriate housing is fundamental. The need for new administrative strategies is underlined in the Commission's Report, including "the higher profile of multidisciplinary programs in the community and within institutional care," as well as ensuring effective and efficient use of resources, ". . . will require the establishment of regional coordinating committees . . ." (Report, 1988). The availability of assessment and rehabilitative services, which should be an essential component of an integrated system of health/welfare care, varies widely in New Zealand. These services are an essential component of a coordinated continuum of care.

The number of disabled in New Zealand has been estimated to be 486,000 (ACC, 1986). This is based on a self-classification system. The Royal Commission challenged the current service delivery system for the disabled: (1) the monocultural approach does not take into account the diverse views on health and illness; (2) the lack of resource sharing reflects a failure to acknowledge the Treaty of Waitangi. "Most disability workers are pakeha and most organizations do not keep records of the race of their clients" (Report, 1988). A move toward active consultation with Maori people was seen as essential.

The Commission noted the multiple discriminations women face in the home and in the workplace. Their current inequitable status can be further affected by ethnicity, disability and age. The statistics demonstrate that women represent the largest number in both the disabled and the elderly categories. Although men are more often disabled by accidents, women are more likely than men to become disabled by illness and they are also "further disadvantaged by the inequality of services provided for illness-related . . . disability." Women most commonly suffer mobility impairment linked to arthritis, which is the most prevalent condition and often an "invisible" disability. "Women over 80 have a 60% chance of being disabled" (Report, 1988). In the current push to short-term hospitalization and in-home care, women are predominantly the care-givers, often without financial remuneration (Croft, 1986).

Strongly linked to these concerns is the lack of current legislation to protect the rights of the disabled. "Disability was not included in the Human Rights Commission Act in 1977 because of paternalistic attitudes and because of fears about the implications, particularly the costs of building modification, lost production and the attitudes of people to a workplace where all employees did not conform to the same image" (Report, 1988.)

The charity ethic is still alive and well in New Zealand, a strength and a weakness in developing comprehensive services. "The 'do-gooder' mentality often disadvantages people within their own organization. Volunteers and staff alike make assumptions about clients which may not be true . . ." (Report, 1988). Not only does the charity ethic affect attitudes, but it is directly related to funding strategies.

> . . . organizations are assuming their responsibilities to educate and inform as well as scrabble over the shrinking charity dollar. But having one's own disability 'sold' in the street in the form of raffle tickets must be a disquieting experience. (Report, 1988)

The theme of empowerment and accessibility is also highlighted in the Royal Commission's Report. "Having a physically accessible environment for all, breaks down barriers to everyday living, in education, recreation, employment, health and other services. Present provisions for physical access are inadequate" (Report, 1988). It is important to note that the report makes the connection between access and special equipment and technology very clear.

Access to an integrated information system for the consumer is an essential prerequisite for any attempt to implement a coordinated scheme. The development of such a system is expensive and complicated, requiring continued commitment to ensure access to relevant and current data. One example of a data base for the consumer and service provider is the bi-annual Manufacturers Guide published by the Disability Information Officers Bureau (DIO, Palmerston North Hospital Board, 1988).

Since 1985, a more specialized network, the New Zealand Association of Disability Information Officers (DIO), has been operating in 11 centres. This is coordinated through the New Zealand Disability Information Bureau, part of the Disabilities Resource Centre in Palmerston North. A number of other phone-lines and associations exist, each providing specific information and/or services, such as the Arthritis Foundation, Samaritans. Statutory bodies, such as the Department of Social Welfare and hospital boards provide a variety of information services as well.

A major problem is the reluctance of the consumers to complain:

> This ambiguity may in part reflect a reluctance to be critical of an item and supplying system on which users have great reliance. (Barnes and Cunniffee, 1986)

If information is not easily accessible, if technology varies in its availability and if the consumer group is timid, a range of responses is, therefore, required to minimize continued discrimination. The consumers of mid-range technology are often reluctant to self-identify due to the stigma of being disabled or growing old. Elderly are often unaware of their disabilities due to the gradual effect aging may have, and they often have the added complication of multiple medical problems. Maori consumers feel like a "minority within a minority" and are noticeably absent from the helping societies and self-help groups. Many are on fixed incomes, so that cost is a major factor.

"Kiwi Ingenuity" or a sense of individual self-reliance and ability to make do is a strongly held value, adding to the reluctance to see technology as a necessity. In many respects, the predominant contribution of technology is still perceived as assisting hospital discharge rate, rather than improving community integration and functioning. Several relevant studies have acknowledged the general medical practitioner's central role in the dissemination of information (Asher et al., 1982; Herman, 1984). This point highlights the need to include general practitioners in any information system, since they are the gatekeepers to health services and resources.

In the present policy for the regionalization of services, there is a danger that a piecemeal approach will further disadvantage the disabled and elderly. The Lottery Board in its research of requests for wheelchair funding, found that hospital boards and area health boards varied regionally in their respective policies and procedures in providing wheelchairs (Lottery Board, 1987). A recent survey on the West Coast demonstrates service delivery problems vary from one small coastal town to another (Stott, 1988). On a national level the only bodies contributing an integrated over-view are in the voluntary sector, the Disabled Persons' Assembly and the Aged Services Council. The recent Law Commission report recommends the establishment of a Minister of Rehabilitation to ensure national coordination is accomplished (Law Commission Report No. 4, 1988).

The major problems facing the disabled and elderly in New Zealand today are as follows: (1) a lack of coordinated and integrated information, (2) inadequate support services, (3) physical access problems, (4) discrimination compounded by racism and sexism, (5) regional differences in the delivery and availability of services, and (6) the lack of national policy and avenues of accountability.

## ERS–LOCALITY STUDY

A detailed study of the "Palmerston North Telephone-linked Alarm System" (Chamberlain & Webster, 1983) evaluates its effectiveness for an "at risk" population of frail elderly in a community of 60,000 people. Living in communities today are a large number of people who are "at risk" in some way, through health and social problems. These include the frail elderly, individuals suffering from specific physical disabilities, individuals susceptible to loss of consciousness and falls. While it is extremely difficult to determine the size of this group, it is known that being "at risk" is correlated with age. In New Zealand today, the proportion of the population aged 65 and over is increasing (Salmond, 1976, p. 20). Combined with this, increasingly sophisticated medical and surgical techniques are aiding the survival of people who may remain "at risk."

In spite of the fact that social practice and economic constraints would be expected to encourage more elderly people to live in the community, this does not appear to be happening. The occupancy rates for residential homes for the elderly are increasing (Taylor, Neale, & Allan, 1981, p. 2), and New Zealand ranks well ahead of some other Western countries with respect to the level of institutional care for the elderly (Shanas, 1971). These results are surprising in view of the fact that it is government policy to maintain and support the elderly as far as possible in their own homes.

Scotts and Koopman-Boyden (1977) also found that this was the preferred living arrangement for most elderly people. Perhaps for these reasons there has been increasing interest in the development of effective and economic means of aiding "at risk'" individuals to remain in their own homes.

## ALARM-CALL SYSTEMS

One solution to this problem has been to provide some form of alarm whereby a person can summon assistance either in an emergency or on a regular basis. The two main criteria for an effective alarm system are: (1) the ability of the person to operate it under emergency conditions to reduce physical harm and discomfort, and (2) the need for a certain and appropriate response to promote security as an aid to independent living.

The study provides a historical overview of the planning and development stages of the ERS. In the development of the referral system, the general medical practitioner was identified as the gatekeeper due to their instrumental role in assessing "at-risk" consumers, earning confidentiality, and sanctioning the technology. The consumers were then assessed by a paramedical community liaison officer to ensure the "most appropriate use of available alarm units." It was estimated 2% of the community's 2,000 elderly living alone would require an alarm, so that 40 units would be sufficient to meet initial requirements.

In 1983, digital equipment manufactured in New Zealand by the Phone Alert Company became available, providing a much needed capability to provide a central monitoring station. This development coincided with a voluntary agency, The Samaritans, establishing 24-hour monitoring services, supplementing friends/relatives/neighbors, and the hospital and police with their own emergency on-call crew.

Since the majority of the consumers for this program would be subsidized through the Disabilities Resource Centre and the number of units would be limited, the following system to prioritize candidates was developed:

A. Physical, Medical, Psychological Factors:
  1. Proneness to falls
  2. Predicted inability to recover from a fall due to weakness, risk of fracture, lack of comprehension, or an inability to respond to unforeseeable endangering situations
  3. Proneness to medical emergency
  4. Fear about their current situation.

B. Social Situation:
 1. If living alone, geographic isolation, dependence on visits from professionals/relatives, and dangerousness of physical environment
 2. If not living alone, but with frail other and/or unattended for varying periods of time
 3. Fear of helpers or relatives about the consumer.
C. Use of Alarm System:
 1. Ability of consumer to comprehend the appropriate use of the system
 2. Physical ability to use the equipment.

The equipment was purchased through fund raising by the Central District Lions Club and ultimate responsibility for the scheme's operation was the New Zealand Disabilities Resource Centre. More recent development of alarm systems reflects the emphasis on "user-pay" as most of the major systems are now commercial operations.

In evaluating the Palmerston North scheme, the demographics of the sample closely align to the national statistics. Eighty-five percent were 65 years or older and 14% were over the age of 85. Eighty-six percent of the clients were women and 69% of these women were widowed. More than half of the consumers (54%) were living alone and a number of the clients suffered from more than one illness. Consumers who were subsidized (rather than private pay) reported appreciably greater difficulty with mobility and stated their health kept them from doing things they liked and impeded activities of daily living.

Consumer attitudes to the alarm system were overall positive. Eighty-three percent rated the alarm as being very important to their lives and easy to use. Installation of the alarms and confidential treatment were satisfactory. Seventy-eight percent felt confident their emergency contacts would be available when necessary and 94% stated their relatives and friends received comfort and "reassurance" knowing they had the alarm system.

## REFERRAL SOURCES

Although 63% of 24 general practitioners contacted were aware of the alarm system and were positive about the scheme, few initiated referrals and their knowledge about the equipment and central monitoring capability was minimal. District health nurses seemed more aware of the scheme and initiated a number of referrals. Restricted mobility and living alone were the major referral criteria, but neither doctors nor nurses listed social isolation, extent of home support and the anxiety of the caregiver as criteria for selection.

## ALARM SYSTEMS

During the ten months of the evaluation, 198 calls were received, 6% were genuine emergencies requiring immediate assistance due to falls or feeling seriously ill. Eighty percent of the calls were due to accidental activation and 14% were due to faults in the equipment. Equipment checks by the voluntary agency were not working satisfactorily and required more technical knowledge and coordination. The Phone Alert equipment was evaluated, using the Canadian Standard for Electrical Aids for the Physically Disabled Persons (Draft CSA Standard Z323.1, 1981). In New Zealand mid-range technology is developed in a variety of ways, not all of which follow conventional routes of safety and reliability testing. The Standards Association of New Zealand (SANZ)-Wellington, Telarc New Zealand-Auckland, and New Zealand Disabilities Resource Centre-Palmerston North are involved in testing and working toward approved standards for equipment. But many products are not formally tested and fall under the "buyer beware" category.

Consumer interviews and discussion with the technical advisors resulted in modifications of the equipment. The central monitoring system operated reliably; the two major periods of inoperation resulted from human error (accidentally turning off the isolating key). Referral and installation of the equipment took between 16-19 days and improvement was needed in coordination of the technical and referring staff.

Overall, the scheme evaluated in 1983 was rated favorably, meeting the emergency needs of "at-risk" individuals living in the community. Since that time, Emergency Response Systems have greatly increased throughout New Zealand and the technology and equipment is vastly improved.

The following table provides some current estimates of the Personal Security Alarm (ERS) Systems being utilized for the elderly and disabled in two centres in New Zealand. There are great regional variations in availability, and these numbers do not designate the percent who are elderly and/or disabled using the units.

Palmerston North:  Population – 62,000

| | |
|---|---|
| Securitas | 80 units |
| Armourguard | 110 units |
| Community Health Services | 40 units |
| (original sample scheme) | |
| Total | 230 units |

Christchurch: Population – 348,172
Armourguard                                    1500 units


## DISCUSSION


An overview of mid-range technology and a locality specific study have been provided as the context for the discussion of the current status of Emergency Response Systems in New Zealand. Despite limited data, it is evident that the changing economic and social climate has fostered a proliferation of companies producing commercial schemes to ensure safety for "at-risk" populations, thus enabling them to remain in their own homes. Whether there are enough units and whether all "at-risk" consumers are able to purchase these systems is not clear. Integration of other services for the frail, elderly and disabled needs to be evaluated to safeguard emergency response systems from being seen as a "cheap" way to discharge people from hospitals instead of providing maximum community integration. Service delivery must meet the vast regional differences in rural and urban communities, especially in rural areas where the lack of competition can result in more expensive and/or limited availability of units. Cultural perceptions of technology combined with personal denial of aging and failing health may affect maximum utilization of various ERS schemes. Continued education and marketing are necessary to ensure appropriate referrals. Safety standards are necessary so that consumers are confident of receiving reliable equipment.

There are numerous positive trends that can be utilized to assist the development of ERS:


1. The Department of Health is developing a nation-wide computer system.
2. Area Health Boards and Social Welfare district devolution will empower local communities to advocate product availability.
3. A proposed federation of disabled information officers would enable a national data base and referral point.
4. The potential commercial value for this product will grow with the changing population.
5. The Royal Commission on Social Policy (1988) stresses the theme of an accessible New Zealand environment that includes the availability of technology.

Perhaps more questions than answers have been raised, but there is the potential for Emergency Response Systems to become an effective technology to assist New Zealand to meet human service needs for the growing cohort of elderly and disabled in the 20th century.

## REFERENCES

Asher, B. et al. (1980). *Wanganui Health Survey.* Dept. of Social Policy and Social Work, Massey University.

Barnes, R. and Cunniffe, W. (1987). *Survey of the Equipment Used and Provision of Services Available to People With Disabilities in the Manawatu Area.* D.P.A. Palmerston North Branch, P.O. Box 143, Palmerston North.

Chamberlain, K. and Webster, Jan (1983). An evaluation of the Palmerston North telephone-linked claim system. *Occasional Papers in Psychology. No. 9.* Massey University.

Croft, Sue (1986). Women, caring and the recasting of need–a feminist reappraisal. *Critical Social Policy,* Summer, 1986.

Disability Information Officers Bureau (1988). *Manufacturers List.* Palmerston North.

Herman, W.R. (1985). The Dannevirke Study: Implications for rural mental health. *Community Mental Health in New Zealand. 1(2).* February 1985.

Hunt, Robyn (1988). People with disabilities. In: *The April Report, Vol. IV: Social Perspectives.* Royal Commission on Social Policy.

Koopman-Boyden, Peggy (1988). Perspectives on the elderly in New Zealand. In: *The April Report, Volume IV: Social Perspectives.* Royal Commission on Social Policy.

N.Z. Law Commission (1988). *Personal Injury Prevention and Recovery.* Law Commission Report No. 4.

N.Z. Lottery Board (1988). *Report on Hospital Board's Criteria for Funding Electric Wheelchairs and Electric Scooters.* NZ Lottery Board, Dept. of Internal Affairs, Wellington. (Unpublished).

Stott, J. (1988). *Report on Survey of Services for the Disability Sector West Coast Region.* Disabled Persons Assembly, P.O. Box 155, Hokitika.

# The Swedish Model
# of Social Alarm Systems
# for the Care of the Elderly

## Bo Stenberg

### GENERAL BACKGROUND

I represent Tele Larm Incorporated, a company owned by the Swedish Telecommunications Administration. My company operates in the whole of Scandinavia and in Switzerland, Belgium, Spain and Austria. We deal mainly in security alarm systems. I am in charge of a business area concerned with emergency response systems for the elderly, the disabled and other frail people.

Tele Larm was one of the first companies to offer equipment and systems to this group of people. In 1978 Televerket Larm, today's Tele Larm Inc., started to develop emergency response systems. The development of these systems has continued ever since, and our present security systems are based on completely new ideas of how the systems must be designed and how they should function.

### Basic Facts

Sweden consists of 284 municipalities. According to our constitution the local authorities and the county council are responsible for social welfare.

Bo Stenberg is affiliated with Tele Larm AB, Sweden.

*135*

*Social Welfare Legislation*

The work of both local authorities and county councils is regulated by legislation. In 1982 the new Social Services Act (Socialtjanstlagen) came into effect. This is a framework legislation which emphasizes the right of the individual to receive municipal services at all stages of his life. Everyone who needs help to support himself in his day-to-day existence has the right to claim assistance if his needs cannot be met in any other way. In 1983 a new Health and Medical Services Act (Halsooch sjukvardslagen) came into effect. According to this Act, health care and medical services shall be available to all members of society, thus ensuring a high standard of general health and care for all on equal terms.

Compared with most other countries, Swedish local authorities and county councils enjoy an unusually autonomous position vis-à-vis the state. Local politicians are directly elected at general elections and both local authorities and county councils levy taxes. The legislation on social services and on health and medical care allow local authorities and county councils very great freedom to plan and organize their own services.

*Care of the Elderly*

We are today very proud of our country and the care of the elderly supplied in Sweden.

The care of the elderly comprises the following main services:

- cleaning (more and more often carried out by cleaning companies)
- cooking (has decreased because of the current trend to distribute convenience food)
- assistance to go to bed/get up
- washing and hygiene
- keeping people company, chatting
- going to banks, etc.
- shopping
- making appointments (doctor, hairdresser, etc.)
- activating
- rehabilitation
- walks

There are three kinds of housing for the elderly:

- private housing (you live in your own home and receive home services help)

- sheltered housing/old-age homes (10-150 people)
- group dwelling (2-10 people)

## The User of Emergency Response Systems in the Care of the Elderly

In Sweden there are 1.5 million people aged 65 and above. Fifty thousand of them have emergency response systems, most of them paid for by the local authorities.

There are also a number of emergency response systems in old sheltered housing units. These old systems (a total of 80,000 units) are now being modernized.

The Swedish market for care phones grows by some 10,000 care phones per year, a figure which is increasing. So is the figure for sheltered housing units where we at present supply 4,000 intercare phones per year.

### Demographic Trends

In January 1989 Sweden had a population of some 8.5 millon. Seventeen point eight per cent of these were over 65 years of age, most of them pensioners. Life expectancy for a newly-born girl was 80.1 years and 74.1 years for a boy.

The number of persons in the age group 65 and above (65+) will not change between now and the year 2000, yet between 2000 and 2020 it is expected to increase by almost 25%. On the other hand, the numbers of the very oldest in the population are continuing to rise, as they have done for some time. The age group 80+ has increased in number by 31% since 1980, with projections showing that between now and the year 2000 the age group 85-89 years is expected to increase by just over 40% and those 90+ by just over 75%.

Age is the single factor which demonstrates the strongest link with consumption of social services and health and medical services. In all probability, therefore, the increase in numbers of the very oldest will be accompanied by a growing burden on the various elements of the services for the elderly.

A government report from 1987 has estimated that staffing requirements will increase by over 70,000 by the year 2000, a staff increase of 80-100%.

The care phone is not meant to replace human care and contact. Consequently, it only complements ordinary care. Since the number of elderly people is increasing, and since it is becoming increasingly difficult to recruit staff, there will be more and more pressure on the economy of local authorities, and the role of the care phone system will continue to increase.

## TECHNOLOGY AND STRUCTURE

As I mentioned earlier, we have three types of housing for the elderly. There are two kinds of emergency response systems to choose between: care phones for private housing and intercare phones for sheltered housing. A combination of systems is used for a group dwelling in accordance with the attitudes and wishes of the local authorities.

### Care Phones

The most common care phone–to my knowledge the only one today–is the auto-dialing type, which automatically dials and connects you with a receiver (see Photo 1). The equipment consists of an attachment unit placed under the ordinary telephone set, an undercarriage, a portable trigger serving as a radio transmitter (in Sweden we use 169 mHz to avoid jamming) and an adapter for the power supply. Our latest model is called TT-90.

The TT-90 can be connected to a standard tone dialing telephone. It has a loudspeaking function, i.e., you can call for help without lifting the receiver. The person who needs help can call for it in three ways: press the red push-button on the attachment unit or the portable trigger (radio) or the connected alarm triggers, if any. Connected alarm triggers are getting more and more unusual since the portable trigger is much easier to bring along, thus offering security wherever you go.

The person who needs help can also use three auto-dialing push-buttons which can be programmed to connect him with members of his family. These push-buttons enable our customers to dial the most frequently used numbers, thereby supplying a channeling of the different kinds of help needed. There is also a green push-button which is used to cancel the call.

Exterior alarms such as fire-alarms can be connected to the TT-90. These exterior alarms used to be connected by means of wire, but we have now developed a fire-alarm with a radio transmitter which makes it very easy to connect. We import this fire alarm from the USA.

Our TT-90 model is sensational because it is self-instructive; it can learn to recognize a certain specific portable trigger. All programming is done by the home help staff via the TT-90 keyboard. After completing

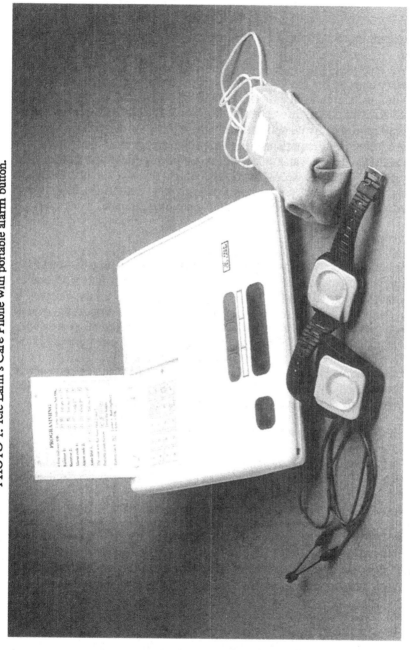

PHOTO 1. Tele Larm's Care Phone with portable alarm button.

programming, the keyboard is covered so as not to distract or confuse the user.

We can program the two receivers that are to be programmed, the primary one and the secondary one. Two receivers are necessary to ensure continuous operation in case of operational failure. All in all, two alarm receivers, two codes, three portable triggers (fire-alarms), three auto-dialing calls and six private numbers can be programmed at a time.

We know from experience that the portable trigger is likely to be exposed to liquids like water, juice, etc., so we have made it water-proof. The top of the TT-90 is water-proof, too, which saves a lot of money by reducing service costs for the users and the local authorities. This is one reason why our TT-90 has been highly and widely praised.

### Function

When somebody needs help he presses either the red push-button of the TT-90 or the portable trigger. The TT-90 then connects him with one or several receivers. When the TT-90 obtains an answer from the receiver, it emits a code telling the receiver who needs help. Depending on the degree of sophistication of the receiver, different kinds of information are available, e.g., medical data. Two-way communication can take place immediately, without any further action from the calling party.

Other people can call the person who has our TT-90 and he can answer the phone call by pressing the portable trigger, i.e., without lifting the receiver. In this case the TT-90 serves as a loudspeaking telephone.

### Intercare Phone Systems

The intercare phone system is similar in function to the TT-90 care phone. The difference is that it operates on an internal network so the user of the security phone does not have to pay for the calls. I will give you an example: we had supplied a sheltered housing unit with 57 flats with care phones, and the newspapers began to write about the fact that the tenants were charged for calling for help. Therefore, the system was replaced by an internal network. Naturally, the security phone also has other advantages: it is, for example, possible to answer a call from any security phone connected to the network when the alarm receiver is left unattended.

### Alarm Receiving

There are two types of receiving systems, apart from private receivers. Both of them can receive calls from the TT-90 as well as from the intercare phone system. The first type is simple and indicates only name and address. The second type is supplemented with a personal computer (see Photo 2).

Care phone receiver stations are continuously manned whereas intercare phone receiver stations are manned from time to time. When they are not manned, pocket beepers make it possible for the staff who are working in the flats to see who needs help and then choose to do either of the following things:

- go direct to the person who needs help
- stay where they are and answer the call for help and talk to the person who calls for help.

When there is an alarm from a TT-90, i.e., an external care phone, the staff in charge of the receiver contacts a nursing team consisting of two persons, by telephone or radio and hands over the mission to them. If the call is an emergency call, an ambulance is sent for.

For external housing, the handling of keys is an organizational problem that we have been working on. We have offered the local authorities a key-handling system. When you are called away to a person who needs you, the keys must be collected and a receipt signed at a central place. When a nursing team goes out, it always has keys. In the countryside, the key can be placed in a keybox outside the house where the person who needs help lives. It is of vital importance that keys are not lost or come into the wrong hands.

### Distribution

So far only local authorities have distributed care phones in Sweden, but lately private companies have started to take over part of the distribution. These companies must be commissioned to do this by the local authorities.

## ECONOMICS

The price of a care phone is between $830 and $1,000. Expenses are borne differently in different local authorities. The costs can be borne by the local authorities or shared by the user and the local authorities. They are never covered by the state, by organizations or insurance. The local

PHOTO 2. Tele Larm's Alarm Receiver Unit integrated with computer with special program.

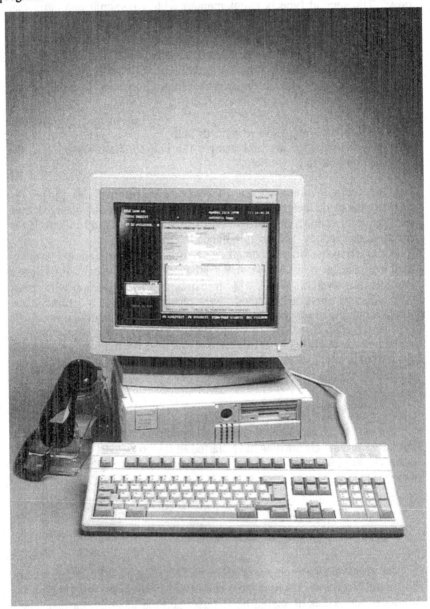

authorities always pay for the care and for costs connected with emergencies.

## *Criteria for Care Phone Users*

The home help staff determines who will receive a care phone. This decision is based on a medical certificate and one of the following criteria must be fulfilled:

- the person has had a myocardial infarct
- the person has problem with his balance
- the person is dependent on a wheel-chair
- the person suffers from dizziness
- the person has other medical reasons
- the person is paralyzed.

## *Care Phone Subscription System*

Since it is difficult for the local authorities to estimate investments and include care phones in their budgets, Tele Larm Inc., in 1988, introduced a care phone subscription system. In the subscription system, the local authorities rent the care phones from us at a fixed monthly fee. The contract is made up for 5 years and the price remains the same throughout the period. The local authorities undertake to buy all the phones they need from us and we offer them a fixed price. Naturally, service is free of charge, so the local authorities pay

- $67 entrance fee
- $20 monthly subscription fee

The advantages for the local authorities are that they

- know their actual costs
- pay no VAT
- have continuous service
- can continuously adjust the number of phones to their needs.

The advantages for us are that we

- have a loyal and regular customer
- can secure long-term cooperation
- can invest in Research and Development.

## OPERATIONS

### Standard Regulations

Today there are no specific standard regulations for care phones, but the European standardization board, SENELEC, is working on it and regulations will come into effect in a year or two. There is also an international standardization board, the IEC, but their work has reached a deadlock. The SENELEC regulations will probably be adopted by the IEC. Economic restrictions are the only restrictions affecting the use of care phones.

### Type and Frequency of Alarms

In Sweden emergency alarm systems are used almost exclusively. In the early eighties passive alarms were also used, i.e., alarms that were activated if no action was registered in a person's flat during a certain period of time, e.g., 8, 10 or 16 hours. This was experienced as supervision, so today there are very few of these passive alarms.

Only 30% of all alarms are emergency alarms. The rest are enquiries or ordinary social calls, etc. Therefore, we have equipped the emergency response system with auto-dialing buttons that connect the user with members of his family or friends.

It is important to be able to distinguish non-emergency calls from emergency calls. As there are various kinds of alarm receiving stations with a variety of emergency response systems connected to them, the number of alarms varies. A station with 2,000 care phone systems connected to it receives 500 alarms per 24 hours and 30% of them are emergencies.

### Integration

At present the TT-90 is not integrated into medical services in Sweden. The TT-90 is, however, always combined with social services and measures. There are always nursing teams to visit the person who needs help.

### User Resistance

There is a certain resistance among users, but also a strong wish and a need to use emergency response services. The reluctance can mainly be explained by the fact that people do not understand the technique and find it complicated. They are scared of what will happen when they press the button. Sometimes they are scared of what this call may lead to (ambulance, etc.) However, the main problem is their fear of the technical aspects. Therefore, the following six considerations have been the lodestar of Tele Larm Inc.:

- enabling the user to stay in his normal surroundings
- enabling the user to feel secure
- taking away the feeling of being supervised
- ensuring as discreet a technique as possible
- enabling the user to call for help in an uncomplicated way
- trying to avoid fixed cable networks.

These aspects are the very basis of the development of today's care phones.

## *Training*

Since the nursing staff employed by the local authorities do not usually have a technical background, they are often reluctant to use some of the techniques applied in their work. This can naturally be explained by a general fear of technical matters and the possibilities or risks that they bring about. In 1986 we began to train personnel and so far we have provided training for some 100 local authorities. The training covers both theory and practice and takes one day. It takes up all the various parts of a care phone system, different models of care phones, alarm receiving, intercare phone systems and pocket beeper systems. A large part of the training is devoted to questions concerning organization, administration and the handling of keys.

Our training has had very positive results. The need for service on our systems has decreased considerably. Many local authorities have chosen to subscribe to training, which ensures a continuous updating of our know-how.

The training of nursing staff in the use of computer-aided receiving systems takes two days. Both the one-day and the two-day training programs are bought by the local authorities.

## BENEFITS OF EMERGENCY RESPONSE SYSTEMS

### *Psychological Benefits*

Several investigations show that, thanks to the distribution of care phone systems, the person who needs help feels more secure and reassured, and he is able to stay in his normal surroundings.

The care phone system has also contributed to family members' feeling more secure–sometimes family members feel so secure and reassured that they tend to visit the person concerned less often.

## Cost Savings

Care in a Swedish hospital amounts to some $300 per day, so you can easily see how economical the TT-90 is. If the TT-90 makes it possible for a person to stay at home, the cost is paid off in three days, and at the same time the hospital care can be offered to somebody who needs it more.

## DEVELOPMENT

At this point, I would like to give you a short review of the care phones which are the result of 10 years of hard development work.

In the seventies, there were emergency response systems consisting of only push-buttons permitting no verbal communication. The development was rather slow.

In the late seventies, however, two Swedish companies started to compete for customers. This was the origin of the care phone systems. It all happened in Malmo, in the south of Sweden.

The two companies were Ericsson and Tele Larm Inc. We were not very successful, mainly because we used fixed cable networks. Therefore, we decided to start from scratch, and in February 1981 we began to develop the new care phone systems. They were dialing systems.

In July 1981 the prototype of the care phone and its receiver was ready. We had 600 care phones made for us, but the demand was so heavy that we had to order another 500 units.

In December 1981 the first phones were delivered. At the same time the development of a new model began, since our customers wanted a slightly different version.

Thus in March 1982 we started the production of 2,000 new units. A total of 6,000 copies were made of this model.

In February 1984 it was time to design a new model, once again in accordance with the wishes and views expressed by our customers. For example, they wanted to have their own keyboard for the unit and they needed to know that the programmed information would not disappear in case of power failure.

A completely new production technique was used, viz. surface mounting. This is the predominant technique in today's electronics industry. Thirty thousand copies were made of this model.

In the fall of 1987 we started the development of a new model of the care phone and its receiver, based on the use of a PC to obtain more and quicker information about the customer or subscriber.

# SCOTLAND

# Community Alarm Systems in Scotland

## Alexander Cameron

### BACKGROUND

In order to set the context for considering the development of community alarm systems in Scotland, some demographic background information will be helpful. Scotland is, of course, part of the United Kingdom but has its own legal and local government structure which differentiate it from the rest of the United Kingdom and which have had a bearing on the way in which services have developed.

The population of Scotland is 5.1 million, of which some 17.5 per cent are of pensionable age. That is to say, women aged 60 plus and men aged 65 plus. This compares with 14.1 per cent of the population who are of school age. Within Scotland there are some marked differences in the proportion of the population which is elderly, with the rural Borders Region having proportionately the largest elderly population at 24 per cent. By the year 2001, the elderly population will increase by 3.4 per cent whilst the over 75s will increase by 15.9 per cent. Of those people aged 65 plus at present, six per cent are housebound whereas 31.4 per cent of those aged 85 plus are housebound.

Scotland therefore has, and will continue to have, a substantial proportion of the population in the elderly age range and will have an increasing-

---

Alexander Cameron is affiliated with Borders Regional Council, Scotland.

*149*

ly elderly population through into the next millenium. Services for elderly people are therefore a very key element in range of Scottish health and welfare services.

The importance of these services is all the more clear when more facts are considered about caring in Scotland. Thirty five per cent of all households have one or more pensioners living in them and 44 per cent of people aged 75 or over live alone. One in 10 Scottish adults are caring for an elderly person. However, the pool of carers is diminishing. In the 1920s, for every person aged over 75, there were 13 people aged between 40 and 60–the age range of most carers. Today the figure is just three. The picture is one therefore of growing numbers of elderly and particularly very elderly people living alone with no family members available to care for them.

Only 1.7 per cent of Scotland's elderly population is permanently in residential care and 2.1 per cent is permanently in hospital care. The very great majority of Scotland's elderly population is therefore living in the community and therefore services which assist and support independence within the community are particularly important and will continue to be so. This is all the more so given the very major structural and legislative change which is currently being planned for as a result of a Government review of care in the community.

Having dealt with the demographic context of Scotland, the structure of welfare services is an important backcloth to the consideration of the development of community alarm systems. Scotland has two tiers of local government, namely, Regional Councils and District Councils but to confuse matters there are also three Island Authorities which combine the functions of Region and Districts. All of these are elected bodies.

The provision of social work services is the responsibility of Regional Councils, each of which has a social work department with wide ranging responsibilities which include the care and protection of children; services for people with disabilities including people with learning difficulties; mental health services; the probation and after-care service for offenders; and services for elderly people. Some 35,000 whole-time equivalent posts are employed in social work departments and in 1988/89 the total net expenditure of social work in Scotland was £403.8 million ($636.6 million).

Responsibility for housing in Scotland lies with District Councils which have responsibility both for the provision of housing and for the strategic planning of housing provision within their area. Alongside the District Councils a substantial amount of public sector housing is provided and managed by the centrally funded body, Scottish Homes, which also provides funding for housing associations which are particularly active in the field of sheltered housing. As far as sheltered housing is concerned, District Councils are responsible for the provision of the buildings while the Regional Councils are responsible for the provision of the warden service. This shared responsibility is a major element in the reason for the development of community alarm systems by Social Work Departments in Scotland whereas the great majority of services throughout the rest of the United Kingdom have been developed primarily by Housing Authorities which have responsibility for both the buildings and the warden services.

The responsibility for Health Services lies with the National Health Service which operates in Scotland through Health Boards which are co-terminus with the Regional Council areas with the exception of Strathclyde Region, the largest of the Regional Councils, which has four Health Boards lying within its area.

## THE HISTORICAL DEVELOPMENT OF COMMUNITY ALARM SYSTEMS WITHIN SCOTLAND

The first community alarm system was established in Central Region in 1979 using radio based equipment with no speech facility. The impetus for the development of the Central Region system came from two factors which were to become common to many systems. Firstly there was the recognition that there was insufficient sheltered housing to meet the needs of a growing elderly population and the curtailment in local government expenditure which was being experienced at that time meant that the supply of places in sheltered housing schemes was not going to keep pace with demand. The question posed by those planning services in Central Region was whether some of the benefits of sheltered housing, namely the warden service and alarm system could be extended to people living in their existing homes. The possibility of this opened up when radio based alarm equipment became available in the United Kingdom in the late 1970s.

The second factor contributing to the Central Region development was the recognition that sheltered housing resident wardens could not be available 24 hours per day. Wardens had been employed on the basis that they would live within the sheltered housing complex, initially with a view to being a "good neighbour." As the elderly tenants of these complexes became more frail then the calls on the "good neighbour" became more frequent and demanding. Most wardens were highly committed individuals who felt a great responsibility to their tenants and who therefore were extremely reluctant to leave the complex in case a call would be made on their alarm system. Increased unionisation of the wardens brought pressure for the appointment of relief wardens but that had the complication of access to the alarm system which usually terminated inside the resident warden's home.

Clearly it was entirely unreasonable to expect resident wardens to be available "on call" on a 24 hour per day, seven day per week basis although it has to be said that that had indeed been the assumption of many people involved in the planning of sheltered housing. Tenants had been led to believe that the warden would always be there to respond to a call on the alarm system. Inevitably there were outcries from relatives when elderly tenants used the alarm and did not receive a response, sometimes for, what at least felt like, several hours. There was a need therefore to provide a means of allowing resident wardens genuine "off duty" time whilst at the same time ensuring the availability of a response to alarm calls. The interfacing of community alarm equipment with the sheltered housing alarm systems could provide a means of achieving this and therefore a further reason for establishing a service had been identified.

The planning of the service within Central Region took some 18 months and drew together representatives from the Health Board and the Housing Authorities. This was a crucial process and one which experience showed required careful and detailed consideration and agreement between the agencies to ensure that the operational practice developed in the best interests of the client. This detailed planning process involving all the relevant parties is one which has not always been followed by other subsequent schemes, with the result that inefficiencies have been built into services from the outset.

The introduction of a community alarm system at that time was the first introduction of new technology into the social service field and as such was an area with which many of those involved in the planning were not familiar. It was important therefore to obtain expert, independent technical advice. This was provided through the Central Government Department which was responsible for radio licencing. Its experts gave advice on the feasibility of the manufacturers proposals and a technical appraisal of the equipment which was being offered.

Again this is an aspect of the planning of services which have developed in the intervening years which has too often been missed with the result that some services have been set up around equipment which is unreliable and inefficient and most worryingly, in some cases, which is not safe. It was not until 1986 that the Research Institute for Consumer Affairs published a comprehensive review of alarm equipment (Dispersed Alarms–A Guide for Organisations Installing Systems R.I.C.A. 1986). In the early days of alarm system development there were many manufacturers offering equipment on the basis of very exaggerated claims as to its effectiveness or indeed its legality. This is less so now since many of these companies have dropped out of the market but the need for good technical appraisal of alarm equipment will always be an important element in system development and planning.

It is perhaps worth raising a concern here at the way in which service providers have responded to the marketing pressures from manufacturers. This has been, and continues to be, a lucrative market and it has therefore been the focus of a great deal of salesmanship, often targeted at elected members of Councils. Systems have been sold as the solution to all problems, often with heavy emotive overtones based on images of elderly people lying for hours on the floor after a fall before being discovered. Councils have therefore been sold the idea of having such a service rather than having identified a service need consistent with their service priorities and having found a means of responding to that need. Alarm systems can all too easily appear to be attractive, "high tech" solutions which seem to be simple and comparatively cheap. Rarely do salesmen provide details of the running costs of equipment or the staffing costs associated with such things as installations or the changing of batteries in remote control units.

Central Region having planned a service which would provide a response to the problems which had been identified therefore set up its Mobile Emergency Care Service using radio based equipment with no speech facility. The service was backed up by mobile wardens who were available on duty 24 hours per day and who, in addition to responding to alarm calls, were involved in routine visiting to all service users. This had the dual function of ensuring that wardens and clients became familiar with each other and of monitoring the well being of the clients, thereby ensuring the early referral on to other services where necessary.

The central monitoring of the alarm system was initially undertaken on Central Region's behalf by Health Board telephonists at a large psychiatric hospital but eventually the use of the system became such that it was necessary to open up a control centre for the service itself although in more recent years this was expanded to provide a control centre function for other out of hours' services of the Council.

The Central Region system is currently in the process of phasing out its radio based alarms which are to become redundant as a result of the changes in regulations arising from the World Administrative Radio Conference (W.A.R.C.). The radio units are being replaced by telephone based equipment with a speech facility. Central Region reports that whereas a large proportion of its clients did not have telephones when the service started 10 years ago, it now finds that the great majority of people referred to the service do have telephones, thereby making the use of telephone based equipment all the more feasible.

Since the implementation of the Central Region system in 1980, every Scottish Social Work Authority with the exception of one of the Island Councils has introduced a community alarm system. Such systems have therefore become an element in the community care strategies of Scottish Social Work Departments. All systems involve some varying degree of partnership with Housing Authorities and all include an interface with sheltered housing alarm systems in their operation. They have been used to augment the services of wardens rather than to replace wardens although there has been a shift away in some areas from having resident wardens, particularly in non purpose-built units.

## CHARACTERISTICS OF THOSE USING COMMUNITY ALARM SYSTEMS

The criteria developed by Social Work Departments have been broadly similar and have focussed on:

a. living alone or having no one in the household capable of providing 24 hour a day support in an emergency;
b. being at risk because of ill health, frailty, disability or extreme anxiety;
c. being unable to summon assistance in an emergency.

Most services indicate that users are likely to be over the age of 75 but none would hold rigidly to this and, indeed, there are examples of services including young children suffering from life threatening illness where parents may have an urgent need to summon help.

All services require some form of assessment before inclusion within their scheme and this is aimed at ensuring that the criteria are met and the service is therefore appropriately targeted. This applies to those people living in their own homes in the community. Sheltered housing tenants are automatically included where their unit is interfaced with the service whether they individually meet the criteria or not.

## TECHNOLOGY AND STRUCTURE

Whilst the initial service described above in Scotland used radio based alarm equipment which had the attraction of very easy installation, it is the case that most Scottish systems are now using telephone based equipment. As the number of homes with telephones installed has increased, particularly amongst the elderly population, this has become all the more possible. The use of a telephone system does however involve a number of costs. Firstly the installation of a suitable socket if one does not already exist and this must be undertaken by British Telecom at an average cost of £41.50 ($70.55) and, secondly, the operating costs of the telephone. In the United Kingdom all calls are chargeable and there is therefore a revenue cost which must be borne either by the service user or by the service itself.

Passive monitoring facilities of alarm systems are rarely used by social work services but increasingly fire alarms/smoke detectors are being connected into systems. This reflects the increased use of such equipment amongst the general population and is a particularly important asset for elderly people who are at high risk of injury from home fires.

For the individual alarm user, the facility of a pendant type remote control unit is particularly important and all services now supply these as a matter of routine.

With regard to the marketing of systems, most social work based services have introduced their own control centres, although a small number of services rely on control facilities provided by other services, most commonly the ambulance service. The operation of control centres which require to be staffed on a 24 hour basis is a significant cost element in the overall running costs of services. This is an aspect which has often been overlooked in the planning of services. A number of services have commenced operation with insufficient staff resources to provide full control centre cover. In particular, service planners and managers have failed to appreciate the amount of routine work which is undertaken by a control centre in programming units into the system, monitoring records, organising changes of equipment, etc. Too often it has been assumed that control centres will only deal with emergency calls and of course these are a very small element in the total traffic which a community alarm service generates.

Within the Scottish context, alarm units are distributed by social work departments based on the current criteria referred to above. This also means that services must have staff available to undertake the installation of units and the removal of units when clients no longer require them. Again this is an aspect of service planning which has too easily been overlooked.

The costs of services are met by Regional Councils through their revenue and capital budgets. No charges are made to clients for the service although where no telephone line exists, clients may be asked to pay for or contribute to the cost of the telephone installation. Most Scottish services make provision for persons who are willing to purchase their own alarm unit to do so and to connect it to the local service at no charge. A feature of the development of a number of services is that they have made use of charitable fund raising to add to the supply of units. Community alarms are particularly attractive for fund raisers since they represent a "good cause" with which the public can readily identify and one in which specific items of equipment can be purchased at comparatively low cost.

## *OPERATIONS*

The fact that services have developed widely and rapidly in Scotland suggests that there is little user resistance to the acceptance of a community alarm service. Indeed, no scheme reports any difficulty in persuading clients to accept the service. There is inevitably some resistance initially but this is usually around the understanding of how to operate the equipment. It is therefore of vital importance that staff spend time explaining how the equipment operates and the circumstances under which it is intended to be used. It is also important that clients understand what happens at the Control Centre and how their calls will be responded to. Opportunities for control centre staff to meet clients face to face are important but often difficult to organise. A simple leaflet explaining the equipment and service and including photographs of control centre staff is valuable both in reminding clients how to operate the system and in helping them to explain to relatives, etc., how it works.

The general experience of services is that clients quickly become reliant on the service and value it highly. Experience has shown that attempts at providing the service on a short-term basis in a crisis often have to be made permanent because of the resistance of clients to do without their alarm unit.

Broadly, three models of response to alarm calls have developed within Scotland:

1. Mobile warden service where wardens are on duty on a 24 hour basis in vehicles and available to respond to alarm calls. In addition, mobile wardens pay routine, regular visits to service users and in some cases may undertake some basic care tasks.
2. Emergency response wardens where a small force of wardens is available to respond to alarm calls where nominated key holders are

not available. In some services these staff are also involved in initial assessments and some follow-up visits. The initial response to alarm calls is however sought from nominated key holders.

3. No response staff but service relies on contact being made with a nominated key holder. Usually services will hold records of at least three nominated key holders. In some cases such key holders can be difficult to identify and substantial amounts of staff time can be consumed in seeking, within local communities, people who are prepared to undertake this function. This is a worrying reflection of the degree of isolation of many elderly people. Services operating on this basis will usually use the police as a last resort fall back response and, generally speaking, this is a function the police are willing to undertake provided the demand is minimal.


### TYPES OF CALLS

There are three major categories of calls which form the bulk of calls to control centres. Firstly, sheltered housing wardens logging off and on site at their units; secondly, fake alarms; and, thirdly, reassurance calls, the dividing line between the latter two being very fudged. It is suspected that many false alarms are generated as a means of testing out the equipment to make sure it is working. It is in fact better if systems encourage their users to call from time to time to reassure themselves that the equipment is indeed operational. Calls for assistance, whether emergencies or less urgent, invariably form the smallest category of calls although, again, it should be noted that this has often not been what is envisaged by those planning services.

The experience of Scottish services is that there is no particularly strong pattern of calls when analysed by time of day. Calls tend to be spread evenly from day to day and there are no major peak times of the day. There tend to be "blips" of activity in the early morning and in the evening, coinciding with people getting up from bed and going to bed. There are times when there is likely to be more increased risk of falling or when people are likely to identify that they feel unwell. Calls in the early hours of the morning are very much less than in day time but are more likely to be calls for help rather than fake alarms.

Good links with medical and social services are important in order to facilitate appropriate responses to calls from control centres. There is some experience of initial resistance from medical practitioners who fear that they may be called frequently by community alarm services and thereby have their workload increased. The usual pattern however is that general practitioners quickly find services to be of benefit to their patients and themselves. Good communication usually develops between control centres and practices with a high degree of trust. General practitioners come to realise that calls from control centres will be important and that operators will have gathered the necessary information to help the general practitioner decide on how he should respond.

## BENEFITS OF COMMUNITY ALARM SERVICES

Within Scotland there has as yet been insufficient research undertaken on the economic benefits of alarm services. There is no sound evidence available that alarm services keep people out of hospital or residential care for instance. What is clear, however, is that there is a high level of satisfaction amongst users of services and in particular most clients report a very much greater sense of security. The importance and value of this should not be underestimated. There is no evidence that the level of contact with informal carers has fallen due to the installation of alarm units.

To maximise their benefits however it is essential that alarm systems are seen as an integral and key element in packages of community care. They must operate on the basis of clearly stated objectives and soundly based assessment. They should become an important element in the range of services available to case managers as new systems of operations come into play within the United Kingdom Social Services.

It seems unlikely that there will be significant changes in the technology other than updating. A wider range of monitoring devices may become available which could open up potential use of systems for supporting people with dementia who at present pose problems for inclusion in services. There are rapidly growing numbers of people who will be the major source of demand on care services in the coming decade. To date, community alarm systems have made no impact on their care but we need to consider ways in which they can. This could for instance be achieved by the use of peripherals to monitor the particular risk of fire or gas escapes or to alert staff to when the confused client has left the house. Such use poses some ethical dilemmas but may have the potential to relieve much anxiety.

# WALES

# Local Authority
# and Housing Association Perspectives
# on ERS in the United Kingdom

Malcolm J. Fisk

## BACKGROUND AND INTRODUCTION

The growth in Emergency Response Systems (ERS) in the United Kingdom has, during the 1980s, been substantial. Whilst accurate statistics (regarding the number of installations) have, to date, been largely absent, we can now estimate that there are some 850,000 households with ERS devices, representing nearly 1,000,000 alarm users (embracing nearly 10% of elderly people). This compares with an estimated 400,000 people in 1981.

The origins of such specialised alarm devices, in the UK, are well documented, having become an essential adjunct of 'sheltered' housing–i.e., that form of accommodation which became fashionable among many housing practitioners during the 1970s and early 1980s. But even within the previous decade it was clear that many grouped dwelling schemes for elderly people incorporated some form of alarm device–a proportion of

---

Malcolm J. Fisk is affiliated with the Reading Borough Council and Rhondda Housing Association, Wales.

*159*

which provided two way speech, albeit to a fixed point (Institute of Housing Managers, 1967).

Sheltered housing has been developed predominantly by local housing authorities. Publically funded housing associations, on the other hand, have played, latterly, an increasingly significant role. The accommodation generally comprises purpose built self-contained apartments for more vulnerable elderly people. Whilst early developments offered, if anything, only simple alarm devices (e.g., bells and buzzers), there was (and remains in all such schemes) a resident 'warden' on hand, at least some of the time, whose role was seen as 'keeping an eye' on the residents and giving occasional help. Her/his job was, and remains, most often described as 'good neighbour.'

In the last decade a growing, though still relatively small, amount of sheltered housing has been built by private developers and increasing sums of private money are now being utilised by housing associations in order to add to their public subsidies. Private developments clearly add to the overall number of ERS users but are outside the scope of this paper.

Whilst sheltered housing has played an important part in accommodating elderly people in the UK, the 'model' on which much of it has been based (derived from a 1969 Government Circular, since scrapped, but including provision for a warden and a 'hard wired' ERS) has increasingly been questioned. Repeated studies, in fact, have pointed out that it is the *quality* of the housing that matters most to the residents and not the warden or the ERS (Butler, Oldman & Greve, 1983; Clapham & Munro, 1988; Oldman, 1989). It is sheltered housing that has, nevertheless, provided the context, in the UK, within which a role for ERS devices was initially recognised.

In parallel with the strong belief (rightly or wrongly) in the merits of sheltered housing, a strong belief in the benefits of ERS has, through this period, developed, and to a large extent remains. Such accommodation has, for instance, been described alternatively as "the greatest breakthrough in the housing scene since the war" (Underwood & Carver, 1979), a "remarkable success" (Eaton, 1980) and "the obvious choice for most elderly people" (Cunnison & Page, 1985). Some researches suggesting that sheltered housing could be provided for most or all elderly people (Heumann and Boldy, 1982) can, however, be contrasted with others advocating the provision of just 50 places per 1000 (Scottish Development Department, 1977).

The need for alternative, and more flexible forms of accommodation to be developed for elderly people has, however, increasingly been strongly argued (Middleton, 1981; Clayton, 1981; Fisk, 1986; Clapham & Munro,

1988). It follows that the benefits of ERS, in this broader context, must be evaluated *on their own merits* and not as an adjunct to the stereotypical and now increasingly discredited model of sheltered housing.

Because of the nature of the accommodation built, however, and in view of the primary role played by housing as opposed to social welfare practitioners in its provision, it was occupied by many for whom there was a housing need but *no additional need* for care or support.

There was (and still is for many local housing authorities and associations), a belief that some kind of 'balance' between less able and more able residents required to be achieved so that the warden would not be overburdened and so that the essentially 'good neighbour' role would not be compromised. The problem was, however, that with some residents 'drifting' into higher levels of dependence, this meant that vacant properties (when they arose) needed to be let to someone who was fit and well and who would not require the additional services (e.g., of an ERS) that came as part of the sheltered housing 'package.'

As a result, the initial emergence of ERS in the UK has reflected a 'property based' approach–the issue of any individual need for care or support often being subservient to housing needs. For a very high proportion of ERS users, in this context, the installation of an ERS has been, therefore, arguably unnecessary.

This tendency towards the property based approach has been exacerbated by virtue of the fact that sheltered housing wardens are generally employed by the housing providers (with exceptions notably in Scotland where the social work authorities have a prominent role). Housing authorities and associations are, needless to say, anxious to restrain their wardens from undertaking 'caring' tasks (except on a very occasional basis) and to avoid incurring additional revenue costs that the latter would suggest.

The sheltered housing 'phenomenon,' it is suggested therefore, diverted attention away from what should have been the main focus in the UK–namely the need to provide good and manageable accommodation within which care and support services could be flexibly proffered and wherein, if necessary, ERS might be provided in response to individual needs. The approach taken can be represented on a continuum (see Fig. 1) the extremities of which represent property based and person (needs) based approaches, the UK perspective being, at least initially, firmly directed towards property.

Belatedly, and following the introduction of individual 'home' ERS units, the approach in the UK is shifting–being increasingly person (needs) based, though remaining significantly less so than is clearly the case in many other countries. The person based perspective also follows increas-

Fig. 1     ERS - THE PROPERTY - PERSON CONTINUUM

Property Based                                         Person Based

I................I................I................I................I

| Grouped | Grouped | Elderly | Needy | Vulnerable |
| dwellings | dwellings | in other | elderly | elderly |
| with | | suitable | not in | with special |
| support | | housing | institutions | needs |

Note: Based on Fisk, 1989.

ing recognition of the shortcomings of sheltered housing (at least in its conventional form) and a predisposition to seek ways of providing services in a more flexible manner. Perchance, however, this British 'anomaly' of sheltered housing has, though discredited, provided a fertile context within which ERS found a sizeable niche and out of which significant technological changes in ERS have materialised.

In the UK we may broadly follow the evolution of ERS from a common origin within those sheltered housing schemes (i.e., stand alone hard-wired systems) along a path which branches with the development of 'home' units for individual dwellings in the wider community (see Fig. 2).

Notable is the rapidity of technological change along both paths–presenting both challenges to the manufacturers (to keep up with their innovating competitors) and to those responsible, in the public sector, for the purchase of ERS. Among the latter remains a high degree of ignorance. Many housing and social welfare practitioners are capable of being 'blinded' by the technology. They are, furthermore, vulnerable to political pressures reflecting the ease by which ERS may be used to facilitate publicising the social credentials of the purchasing body.

The market has been (and will remain to a certain extent) essentially market led. Forthcoming innovations (e.g., possibly relating to voice activation, body monitoring, etc.) may have a further dramatic effect on the UK ERS market. The acceptability of such ERS devices, however, will, require (as it does now) that the personal privacy of ERS users is not compromised and that any damaging psychological consequences (e.g., reduction in motivation for self care) are avoided.

The home ERS unit has, arguably, heralded a period wherein hard wired systems in sheltered housing or grouped dwellings will play a di-

Fig. 2    EVOLUTION OF ERS IN THE UNITED KINGDOM

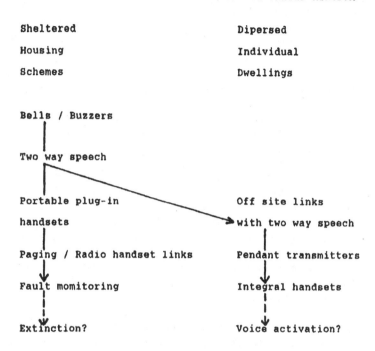

Sheltered                           Dipersed

Housing                             Individual

Schemes                             Dwellings


Bells / Buzzers

Two way speech

Portable plug-in                    Off site links

handsets                            with two way speech

Paging / Radio handset links        Pendant transmitters

Fault momitoring                    Integral handsets

Extinction?                         Voice activation?

minishing role. It has, for instance, enabled provision, by local authorities (whether with housing or social welfare responsibilities), on more clearly person based rather than property based criteria. It has, furthermore, facilitated the emergence of a broader concept of sheltered housing that has been termed 'sheltering in your own home'–i.e., not requiring the elderly person to move to any specialist form of accommodation. And, notwithstanding the fact that many elderly people will still be living or may wish to live in 'grouped' forms of housing (sheltered or not), the cost of 'home' ERS units is now closer to the unit cost of devices installed in such grouped contexts.

## *LOCAL AUTHORITY AND HOUSING ASSOCIATION PROVISION OF ERS*

The increase in the number of 'home' ERS units has, in the past 2-3 years been dramatic. To illustrate the point, in 1988 residents in sheltered housing and grouped dwelling schemes for elderly people represented some 70% of alarm users but now comprise just an estimated 55%. This is despite an increase in the absolute number of 'hardwired' ERS from some 500,000 to approximately 550,000 and complements an exponential growth in the number of users of 'home' ERS units as

a. sheltered housing and grouped forms of accommodation become less favoured options, and

b. social welfare, health authorities and other agencies (voluntary or private) become more widely involved in ERS provision.

Local authorities (essentially housing) are still (at 31st March 1990) by far and away the most important providers of ERS (see Fig. 3) as reflected in the number of central controls they operate–though other agencies are taking a more prominent role. Of the 301 central control facilities in the public sector, for instance, 274 are operated by District, Borough or Islands Councils, in almost all cases being run by the Housing Departments of those authorities.

Social Services/Work Authorities have only a subsidiary role, with the notable exception in Scotland where 8 out of the 20 central controls are operated by them. Health Authorities are notably absent though this obscures the fact that many (notably in Scotland) have made capital and revenue contributions to assist the establishment and operation of such controls. Housing Associations operate 15 central controls, four of which have been transferred from local authorities under provisions embodied within recent legislation.

In Wales, as can be noted, there are 16 public sector central control facilities of which three are operated by social services authorities. The situation is complicated by planned legislative change, much of which is emerging out of comprehensive reviews of the way in which care and supportive services are provided in the United Kingdom. Some of the legislation has direct implications for future ERS provision by virtue of the tightening of the financial constraints within which such schemes have been traditionally funded.

Important portents of the changes were made clear from two reviews published in 1988. Both were commissioned by the Secretary of State for Social Services. The first was undertaken by Sir Roy Griffiths with terms of reference to "review the way in which public funds are used to support community care policy and to advise . . . on the options for action." The second, undertaken by a Committee chaired by Lady Gillian Wagner, had the remit to "promote a fundamental change in the public perception of the residential sector and of its place in the spectrum of social care."

Both reviews embraced common strands that endorse much that was, and remains, central to UK Government thinking–i.e., seeking to maximise the possibility of the care of needy groups (notably vulnerable elderly people) in the community rather than in institutional forms of accommodation *and* seeking to improve the targeting of resources (thereby effecting better value for public money). These themes are further endorsed in the Government's own response to the reviews and given expression in their 'Caring for People' White Paper published in 1990.

In the housing, rather than caring, context legislative change has, however, already taken place. This has tended to systematically restrict future options for housing services and promises (per the recommendation in the Griffiths Report) to concentrate the focus of attention of housing authorities on 'bricks and mortar' rather than care provision. Of particular note is the 1988 Housing Act which provides the mechanism whereby the transfer of housing functions to, e.g., housing associations, is facilitated. It requires, furthermore, 'economic' rents and services charges (i.e., without additional subsidy) to be levied for housing 'services.'

Already the legislation has had an impact on significant numbers of local housing authorities who have transferred or plan to transfer their public housing stock to housing associations. Of the four authorities which had succeeded in such transfers before 31st March 1990, it is interesting to note that all operated central control facilities. These were included in the transfers and are now operated by the derivative housing associations. No such transfers have taken place in Wales.

The manner of local authority and housing association provision is complex and variable. Many central control facilities provide monitoring services for other agencies and accept private subscribers. The scope for further central control installations will become, therefore, increasingly restricted–though there is substantial room for growth in the number of ERS users linked to each central control facility.

Given the current legislative context, the impact of recent reviews, and the rapidity of technological development, it is clear that the moves towards a more person based approach to ERS provision are likely to accelerate. Local housing authorities will play a relatively diminishing role as the scope for ERS is explored more fully by social welfare and health professionals. To the latter, housing associations, rather than local housing authorities, may appear to be the more ready partners in any collaborative arrangements.

Indeed, many housing associations (especially those of larger size) are beginning to develop more substantial roles in relation to the care and support of elderly people. Some are actively seeking, not just to proffer

Fig. 3   CENTRAL CONTROL FACILITIES OPERATED BY LOCAL AUTHORITIES
AND HOUSING ASSOCIATIONS IN THE UNITED KINGDOM

|  | Wales | England | Scotland | N.Ireland | Total |
|---|---|---|---|---|---|
| District, Borough and Islands Auth. | 13 | 252 | 9 | 0 | 274 |
| Social Services/ Work Auth. | 3 | 1 | 8 | 0 | 12 |
| Housing Assoc. | 0 | 11 | 3 | 1 | 15 |
| Total Public Sector | 16 | 264 | 20 | 1 | 301 |

Notes:

1) Central control facilities of any local authority or housing
association can comprise more than one receiver device.
Increasing numbers of such facilities, in fact, incorporate the
equipment of several manufacturers, in some cases such equipment
being linked to a single computerised data base.

2) With few exceptions, the equipment installed offers two way
speech (albeit that the direction of speech is controlled by the
central control operator).

3) The central controls enumerated in the table are those which
link or plan to link 100 or more clients (i.e. excluding ERS
confined to sheltered housing schemes and some others installed
for local management reasons).

4) To the enumerated central controls might be added an estimated

40 such facilities in the private and voluntary sectors,
suggesting that at 31st March, 1990, there was an overall total
of circa 340 central control facilities in the UK.
5) Housing Associations are included as public sector bodies
despite the small (albeit increasing) usage of private monies to
help fund both sheltered housing developments and ERS
installations.


'bricks and mortar' but also to act as agents for social welfare authorities in the provision of care and support services. The number of housing associations with central control facilities are, therefore, expected at least to double, and double again in number over the next 2-3 years–with social welfare and health authority roles also becoming more prominent.


## PERCEPTIONS OF ERS

The manner of evolution of ERS in the UK, being essentially property based and 'rooted' within local housing authorities rather than housing associations, has resulted in a perception of the role of ERS that is likely to be distinctly different from that which has emerged in other countries. The 'standard' facilities of ERS in sheltered housing, for instance, whilst incorporating from an early date, two way speech, have almost invariably omitted passive and/or activity monitoring functions. The need for such 'extras' (as they are perceived) has rarely been considered in the UK context . . . after all, with the presence of a warden living close at hand, there would normally be a daily check on the wellbeing of residents and, therefore, arguably *no* possibility of someone falling ill, or dying, without being discovered for any extended period.

Even with the sudden expansion of ERS (by virtue of the use of 'home' units), local housing authorities and housing associations in the UK have still not awakened to the potential of passive/activity monitoring. Home ERS units, therefore, whilst sometimes incorporating *provision* for passive or activity monitoring are normally confined to usage in *precisely the same way* as ERS in the sheltered housing context. The only real exception to the normal pattern of usage is the provision of pendant (or less commonly, clip-on or wrist watch type) transmitters as triggering devices as opposed to hard-wired pull switches characteristic of sheltered housing or groups of dwellings.

As the emphasis moves to a person based approach, so there will be increasing attention on assessing individual needs. Clearly such assessment, as housing authorities confine themselves to a 'bricks and mortar' role, will be undertaken by social services/work (and, perhaps health) authorities and will require that the potential of passive and activity monitoring functions is properly considered. Such consideration will, furthermore, require to consider carefully the role of ERS within the overall framework of 'care in the community.' It is to be hoped that whilst ERS expands to meet the needs of a wider range of elderly clients (and where the investment of public money is made) it will be seen to be better targeted and more likely, therefore, to maximise the benefit to the ERS users.

## *TECHNICAL ISSUES FROM A USER PERSPECTIVE*

Already, to be fair to local housing authorities who have pioneered the use of ERS in the UK, dramatic improvements have been made as a result of user pressure–both in terms of the reliability and versatility of equipment and in terms of cost competitiveness. Pressure by such authorities (supported and stimulated by various pieces of research, most notably that undertaken by the Research Institute for Consumer Affairs and, more recently, by the British Standards Institution), have resulted in a plethora of safeguards relating to performance and safety. Manufacturers unable to meet increasingly demanding user specifications have disappeared from the marketplace such that ERS in the United Kingdom is now the preserve of essentially 6 contenders. Their share of the UK (public sector) central controls market amounts to 96.3% and is shown below (Fig. 4).

Notable is the strong position of Tunstall Telecom whose presence in the ERS marketplace is also becoming prominent outside the United Kingdom (see Photos 1 and 2).

The nature of the UK marketplace is such that a substantial part of the debate about ERS has focussed on issues of the compatibility of equipment (the need being argued to avoid manufacturer monopolies) rather than the intrinsic benefits or disbenefits of ERS in relation to the care needs of elderly people. Significant, therefore, is the increasing compatibility of ERS equipment in the UK.

Over 50 central control facilities have taken advantage of this greater flexibility and most others now have the option of buying equipment from

Fig. 4    ERS MANUFACTURERS/SUPPLIERS  --  UNITED KINGDOM CENTRAL

CONTROL (PUBLIC SECTOR) MARKET SHARES


| | | |
|---|---|---|
| Tunstall Telecom | 213 | 57.0% |
| Shorrock | 46 | 12.3% |
| Modern Vitalcall | 37 | 9.9% |
| Davis | 28 | 7.5% |
| Cass | 20 | 5.3% |
| Wolsey | 16 | 4.3% |
| Homelink | 4 | 1.1% |
| Oakland | 4 | 1.1% |
| ANT | 3 | 0.8% |
| Others | 3 | 0.8% |
| TOTAL | 374 | 100.0% |


Notes:

1) Some suppliers of ERS include equipment manufactured by their
competitors. The tabulation refers, therefore, to the supplier
of the receiving equipment installed at central control
facilities.

2) The total is higher than the number of central control
facilities on account of increasing numbers of such locations
having multiple receiving devices installed.

multiple sources. Fig. 5 shows, through use of an 'index of diversity' (i.e.,
the number of alternative equipment sources known to have been tapped),
the extent to which this has been done.

The impetus for this has undoubtedly resulted from the intensity of the
debate on compatibility, much of which has highlighted the need for
public authorities to be accountable for their spending. One Welsh author-

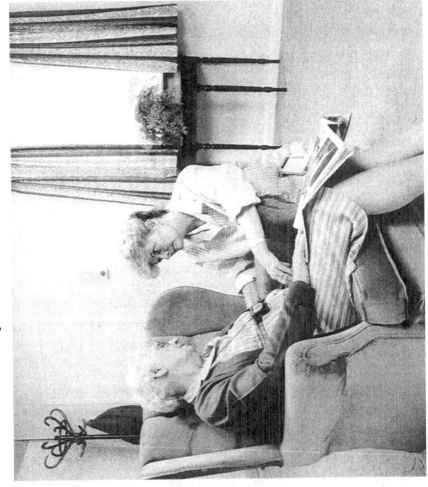

PHOTO 1. Piper Haven Unit by Telecom–Warden responds to call.

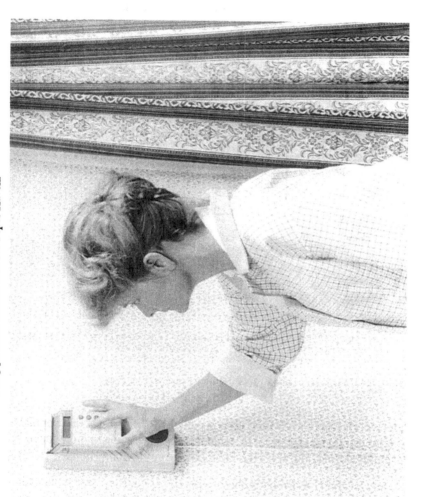

PHOTO 2. Warden using portable control unit for Piper Haven.

Fig. 5    ERS INDEX OF DIVERSITY FOR UNITED KINGDOM CENTRAL CONTROL

(PUBLIC SECTOR) FACILITIES

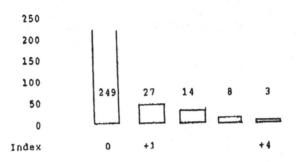

Note:

The index is derived by subtracting the number of 'points of

contrcl' at a central control facility from the number of types

(manufacturers) of equipment linked to that facility.  It shows,

therefore, the extent to which central control facilities have

benefited from increasing equipment compatibility.

ity, Newport, which for a long time installed ERS from just one supplier, has demonstrated a high level of awareness of the issue and more recently has sought to break out from the monopoly, arguing that (Thomas, 1989)

> any customer of a monopoly supplier needs constant reassurance that their interests and the interests of the elderly person *and* thc local ratepayer, are being taken into account.

In Newport's case a second receiver device has now been installed. In other instances various 'interfaces' have, instead, been developed– some 52 of the central controls enumerated in Fig 3 interfacing (in some manner) the equipment of more than one manufacturer (where either different receivers are linked to a common computerised data-base–what has been described as a 'hybrid' configuration, or equip-ment installed in the home is linked, via the medium of telephone or radio, to the receiver of another manufacturer–the 'ideal' configura-tion).

The demise of such interfaces has, however, been heralded by the imminent emergence of a 'National Signalling Protocol' (NSP) to which most main manufacturers are now committed. Local authorities and housing associations will, in this context, be increasingly able to 'mix and match' their equipment–getting the best deals from the manufacturers and thereby maximising value for public money. It will, furthermore, strengthen the bargaining position of ERS users and give scope to smaller equipment manufacturers to enter the market.

The NSP is to be enshrined in a new British Standard (anticipated in 1991) which, though not mandatory, is likely to be insisted upon by a growing number of buyers. The issue of protocols remains, at the time of writing, one that still remains to be considered in the equivalent European context (Cenelec)–but wherein it is possible that the NSP will be adopted at least by other countries of the European Community.

Such protocols, of course, relate to ERS operating via the public telephone network. These represent a clear majority (93%) of systems installed in the UK, the dominance of which is considered likely to continue.

## CONCLUSION

The pattern for local authority and housing association use of ERS in the United Kingdom is set, being largely determined by the emergence and initial usage within sheltered housing schemes. It is now characterised, however, by

i. the shift from a property based to a person (needs) based perspective with better targeting of resources;

ii. the increasing role of social services/work authorities, health authorities, and housing associations;

iii.the increasingly confined role ('bricks and mortar' only) for local housing authorities;

iv. the potential for greater usage of activity and passive monitoring devices.

v. the increasing potential (by virtue of the introduction of a National Signalling Protocol) for equipment compatibility.

The UK shares, however, with most other nations experiencing the growth of ERS, the need for more research into the sociological and psychological effects of the new technology. Some of the North American studies have, for instance, pointed to certain dangers and disbenefits, albeit to only a minority of ERS users (Sherwood and Morris, 1981; Lerner and Stevens, 1986). Some British work is commencing at the University of York, and addresses some of the issues–but the rapidity of development of ERS technology demands that more work must be done and that there must be cross frontier collaboration between researchers.

The changes that are taking place in the UK, however, are within a context where there are now

a. better safeguards for the ERS equipment purchaser and user; and
b. increasing opportunities to apply ERS technology more effectively and flexibly.

Local authorities and housing associations in the United Kingdom are, therefore, in a position to target resources more effectively and thereby, to obtain better value for public money.

## REFERENCES

British Standards Institution (1986) *Recommendations for Social Alarm Systems,* BS 6804.
Butler, A., Oldman, C., and Greve, J. (1983) *Sheltered Housing for the Elderly: Policy, Practice and the Consumer,* George Allen and Unwin, London.
Clapham, D. and Munro, M. (1988) *A Comparison of Sheltered and Amenity Housing for Older People,* Central Research Unit Paper, Scottish Office, Glasgow.
Clayton, S. (1981) "Sheltered Housing, an Intensive or Extensive Service?" in *Health and Welfare Services for the Elderly: Initiatives in the 1980's, Occasional Paper in Health and Welfare No. 1, Department of Social Administration, University of Lancaster.*
Cunnison, S. and Page, D. (1985) *For the Rest of their Days, Humberside College of Higher Education,* School of Applied Social Studies, Hull.
Eaton, J.H. (1980) "Sheltered Housing: Another Concept," *Housing,* April.
Ewen, I. and Fisk, M.J. (1989) "Technical and Practical Issues in Alarm System Development," in Fisk, M.J., (Ed) *Alarm Systems and Elderly People,* The Planning Exchange, Glasgow.
Fisk, M.J. (1984) "Community Alarm Systems: A Cause for Concern" *Housing Review,* Vol. 33, No. 1, Jan/Feb.
Fisk, M.J. (1986) *Independence and the Elderly,* Croom Helm, London.
Fisk, M.J. (Ed) (1989) *Alarm Systems and Elderly People,* Planning Exchange, Glasgow.
Griffiths, R. (1988) *Community Care, Agenda for Action,* HMSO.
Heumann, L. and Boldy, D. (1982) *Housing for the Elderly,* Croom Helm, London.

Institute of Housing Managers (1967) Grouped Dwellings for the Elderly.

Lerner, J.C. and Stevens, A.B. (1986) "Personal Emergency Response Systems," Background Paper No. 3, The Commission on Elderly People Living Alone, Baltimore.

Middleton, L. (1981) *So much for So Few: A View of Sheltered Housing*, Institute of Human Ageing, University of Liverpool.

National Institute for Social Work (1988) "Residential Care: Report of the Independent Review" (chaired by Lady Lillian Wagner), HMSO.

Oldman, C. (1989) "The Role of Housing in Community Care," *Generations– Bulletin of the British Society of Gerontology*, No. 11, Autumn.

Research Institute for Consumer Affairs (1986) *Dispersed Alarms*, London.

Scottish Development Department (1977) *Scottish Housing Handbook 1: Assessing Housing Needs–A Manual of Guidance*, HMSO, Edinburgh.

Sherwood, S. and Morris, J.N. (1981) "A Study of the Effects of an Emergency Alarm and Response System for the Aged," Hebrew Rehabilitation Center for the Aged, Boston.

Thomas, C. (1989) "Case Study 1: Newport Borough Council" in Fisk, M.J. (Ed) *Alarm Systems and Elderly People*, The Planning Exchange, Glasgow.

Underwood, J. and Carver, R. (1979) "Sheltered Housing," *Housing*, Mar/Apr/ June.

# ENGLAND

# Alarms and Telephones in Emergency Response– Research from the United Kingdom

Anthea Tinker

## INTRODUCTION

There is no doubt about the interest in alarms in the United Kingdom (UK). Articles in journals, conferences and advertisements increasingly focus on the contribution that alarms can make to enabling elderly and disabled people to live at home. There are a number of reasons for this. First there is overwhelming evidence that most elderly people wish to remain in their own homes and not move to an institutional setting (e.g., Tinker, 1984b). There are also some indications that the older they are the more pronounced becomes this desire (Salvage, 1986). Second there are developments in home care options, including alarms, which make this possible. Third, there are demographic pressures. Although numbers of elderly people will only increase by about half a million by the end of the century in the UK nearly all that increase will take place among the very elderly, i.e., the over 75s. The number of elderly people living alone is also

Anthea Tinker is affiliated with Age Concern Institute of Gerontology, England.

*177*

expected to increase. Fourth there is extensive advertising by manufacturers aimed at public and private providers of care, such as local authorities, but also at elderly people and increasingly at families. A recent fairly typical advertisement said "Peace of mind for the whole family." Whether there is an equal amount of interest by elderly people themselves will be discussed in this paper.

This paper will concentrate on elderly people but obviously many of them will have disabilities. It also has to be noted that the research on which this paper is based covers not only people who live alone but others as well. However, while about 30% of elderly people live alone in the UK, in schemes with alarms covered by the research between two thirds and three quarters lived alone. What I propose to do in this paper is to look briefly at the following with a focus primarily on alarms but bringing in telephones where appropriate:

- the history and background
- the research on which this paper is based
- evidence about coverage
- use
- benefits
- problems
- costs
- conclusions.

The main focus of the paper is evidence of the experiences and views of elderly people. Technical aspects of alarms and management issues will be mainly dealt with by colleagues.

## HISTORY AND BACKGROUND

No one has written a definitive history of alarms in the UK but there is no doubt that their origins lie in the development of sheltered housing. Sheltered housing, often called congregate housing in other countries, is grouped housing (flats or bungalows) where elderly people live independently with some communal facilities, a warden and an alarm system to which she responds as a good neighbour. Schemes like this have been increasingly developed by local authorities and housing associations since the 1950s (nb a housing association is a non profit making voluntary body formed to provide housing).

Sheltered housing developed rapidly in the public sector after a government circular (Circular 18/57 *Housing of Old People*) encouraged them.

(See Tinker, 1984a for a detailed account of their subsequent development.) Sheltered housing has been increasingly provided in the private, for profit, sector since about the beginning of the 1980s.

Dispersed alarms, that is alarms for people in their own individual homes rather than in grouped dwellings, began to be provided in the late 1970s. They were often based on a sheltered housing complex and the alarm scheme was extended to homes in the neighbourhood. Central control centres then began to be set up, partly so that wardens in sheltered housing could go off duty and someone else could answer the alarm, and partly so that one of the benefits of sheltered housing could be extended to people in their own homes without them having to move.

This emphasis in keeping people in their own homes has always been a feature of policies in the UK. Community care policies are both to enable people to stay in their own homes and as part of a policy to transfer people out of institutions. The UK already has one of the lowest rates of people in institutions (hospitals, nursing homes and old people's homes) in the world. Only about 5% live in institutions and approximately a further 5% live in sheltered housing. The recent government White Paper *Caring for People: community care in the next decade and beyond* (Department of Health, 1989) listed as one of its key objectives "to make proper assessment of need and good case management the cornerstone of high quality care. Packages of care should then be designed in line with individual needs and preferences" (p. 5). Alarm systems are mentioned among the adaptations which can be provided (p. 25).

Dispersed alarms are mainly provided by local authorities and housing associations for their own tenants but sometimes elderly people in the private sector are allowed to buy into the system. There are also some solely private schemes where the alarm has to be bought and then a service charge paid to subscribe to a control centre, either a private or a public one.

This paper is concerned with alarms that give an emergency response to the individual person who activates it themselves. It does not cover alarms that can be activated by a condition (e.g., high blood pressure, heart conditions, etc.). Body monitoring raises all kinds of different issues although some, such as confidentiality of centrally recorded information, applies to all kinds. Some of the alarm systems I shall talk about do have environmental monitoring devices such as smoke or fire detectors.

## THE RESEARCH ON WHICH THIS PAPER IS BASED

There have been two main studies of *dispersed alarms*. The first is a study for the Department of the Environment (DOE) of innovatory ways of enabling elderly people to remain in their own homes *Staying at Home: helping elderly people* (Tinker, 1984b). After national surveys of different kinds of innovations to enable elderly people to stay in homes of their own it was decided to evaluate two different kinds. The first was home care schemes, such as intensive domiciliary help or paying a neighbour, and the second was different kinds of communication schemes involving either alarms and/or telephones. Personal alarm systems were not widely in use at this time but two schemes were included. The alarm systems in this research included one based solely on the telephone. This was an Emergency Telephone Information Service. There was a 24 hour telephone control point for people to ring in an emergency and for regular calls to be made to clients. The purpose was both for emergency use and to keep regular contact with clients. The research took place between 1981-82. After national surveys of local authorities a representative number were chosen for detailed evaluation. This included interviewing the providers and other agencies, a sample of 1,310 elderly people and 251 members of staff.

The second was a study of dispersed alarm systems (Research Institute for Consumer Affairs (RICA) 1986). This, too, had national surveys and interviews with 369 elderly and disabled people. There were two main differences between the pieces of research. The study on innovatory schemes included costs and the RICA study included a technical appraisal of schemes. This was later updated and appeared in a Consumers's Association Journal *Which* (*Which* November 1989). Most other research is of local schemes but these too can be valuable (e.g., Butler and Oldman, 1981, McGarry 1985, Fisk, 1989).

The most recent research on telephones was an exploratory study, *The Telecommunication Needs of Disabled and Elderly People* (Tinker, 1989a). It was undertaken for the Office of Telecommunications, OFTEL, and included individual interviews with 100 disabled and elderly people and group discussions.

There is also evidence from research on sheltered housing. The only national survey was undertaken in the late 1970s (Butler, Oldman and Greve, 1983). This included interviews with 608 elderly people and 248 wardens. However, this research is now twelve years old and must be treated with caution as alarms have developed greatly since then. There has been other, more recent research, in Scotland which covered 496 tenants in 12 schemes run by local authorities and housing associations (Clapham and Munro, 1988). And others have looked at particular providers, e.g., Anchor housing association (Fennell, 1986). In addition research has just been published on very sheltered housing (Tinker, 1989b). This is sheltered housing with extra care, usually the provision of 24 hour wardens, help with domestic and personal tasks for tenants and the provision of meals. This was a national study in England and Wales of both local authorities and housing associations. As well as interviews with providers and other agencies, a sample of 1089 elderly people and 421 staff were interviewed and costings carried out.

## EVIDENCE ABOUT COVERAGE, TYPE AND USE OF ALARMS

*Coverage*

National figures for numbers of people with alarms are not available in Great Britain and this is in itself interesting. Even in a recent (1984) survey of disability the only information available is that three per cent of all disabled adults had a personal alarm defined as "a gadget to summon help" (Martin, White and Meltzer, 1989). The two major studies of alarms (Tinker, 1984b, RICA, 1986) did not quantify provision. However, in 1985 the RICA study found that in the United Kingdom 43 per cent of social services and 62 per cent of housing departments operated alarm systems but numbers of clients varied (RICA, 1986 and Personal Communication). It is also known that about 5% of elderly people live in sheltered housing and nearly all of them will have an alarm.

More is known about the extent of telephone coverage. In 1985 in Great Britain 83 per cent of the population had a telephone (Office of Population Censuses and Surveys (OPCS), 1989). This contrasts with 78 per cent for all households containing at least one elderly person aged 65 and over and 69 per cent for an elderly person living alone.

*Type*

Most sheltered and very sheltered housing has fixed alarms with pull cords or push buttons in different locations in the home. Many of these are now being replaced by personal alarms. Many of the dispersed alarms in the 1984 study were also activated by pull cords or push buttons but there were two schemes with personal alarms of the pendant type. The RICA study shows that dispersed alarms are more likely to be allocated to people at higher risk and with a greater incidence of emergencies than those in sheltered housing.

The kinds of dispersed alarms that are available can be classified under the heading of who responds. They are alarms:

- with no formally organised response (i.e., a flashing light outside the building–of very limited value)
- to a warden or neighbour in the community
- to a warden in sheltered housing
- to a member of staff in an old people's home
- to a central control point where the respondent might be a relative, neighbour, friend or a professional member of staff such as a community nurse.

Details about all these kinds of schemes are given in the 1984 study. It is interesting to note that attention is turning very much to the use of community resources, such as a common room, in the public sector. This is all part of the emphasis on the more intensive use of sheltered housing and old people's homes by a wider group of people.

## Use

Most research studies show that large numbers of people never use their alarm or had not used it in the last year. For example figures for those who had not used their alarm in the last year were 67% in the *Staying at Home* study, 62% in very sheltered housing and 81% in sheltered housing. In the *Staying at Home* study more people had used the personal alarm. Very dependent elderly people and those living alone were most likely to have used the alarm but not necessarily more frequently. Many people only use the alarm once during the year. For example in the *Staying at Home* study of elderly people with an alarm who had used it in an emergency 45% has used it once, 48% between two and five times and 7% more than five times.

Most research also shows that the majority of calls are not genuine emergencies. False alarms due to technical faults appear to be comparatively rare, apart from the teething period after installation. Alarms set off by mistake by the elderly person or visitor are more common. Then come the non emergency calls which range from requests for some kind of help to someone wanting to chat. The single most important use for the alarm was for emergencies. Forty-one per cent of those with alarm schemes in the *Staying at Home* study have used it for this purpose. Of these people 46% had had a heart attack/stroke/collapsed or were taken ill and 39% had fallen. It is striking that one third of elderly people with the personal alarms had had an emergency and had used the alarm the previous year.

Emergencies had occurred at all times of the day and night with most at night. For elderly people with an alarm and using it for an emergency the *Staying at Home* study showed that 37% had used it at night, 25% in the morning, 22% in the evening and 16% in the afternoon. Overall 16% of those with an alarm had used it at night (but half had used it only once)–all had been taken ill or had a fall.

Alarms then did have an important role to play, especially for emergencies and at night.

The main use of the *telephone* by the elderly and disabled people who were interviewed in the OFTEL study was for emergencies. It is interesting that a telephone was rated higher than neighbours. An alarm might have met the needs of some of the group who wanted to contact someone in emergencies but probably only in addition to a telephone. This is because of the role of the telephone for social reasons–mainly keeping in touch with relatives. It is significant that over a quarter of the sample rated the emergency use as of equal importance to the social use.

Telephones are not as versatile as alarm systems but are cheaper. Even if extension points are available elderly people are unlikely to be able to reach them if they fall. An alarm system operated through the telephone is probably ideal. Nevertheless the telephone does have the advantage of people from outside being able to use it to keep in touch with the elderly person.

## BENEFITS

There appear to be three kinds of benefits from alarms. One is getting a response to a particular need whether this is for an emergency or a request for services. The second is that of reassurance. The third is keeping in touch with the outside world. Looking at these in turn most people do seem to get the immediate response they need.

For those with an emergency 89% in the *Staying at Home* study said that they got all the help that they needed. Nearly everyone in the very sheltered housing study said that they were given all the help they wanted when they used the alarm. As we have seen most of the emergencies involved people falling. A quick response can mean that they can be found and action taken promptly.

Turning to reassurance the RICA study pointed out that, although alarms may be used for situations which are not genuine emergencies "such use does not necessarily detract from the value of the service as it provides both reassurance and an opportunity to become familiar with the system" (RICA, 1986, p. 6). The reassurance point is relevant too to critics who point to the high proportion (about 40 per cent in each study who had not used the alarm in the last 12-18 months). Although there is little research on informal carers of elderly people who have alarms it is a reasonable assumption that they too have a sense of reassurance and peace of mind when their relative has an alarm.

Keeping in touch with the outside world is a third element in alarms. This is less easy to accommodate with an alarm system whose main purpose is to respond to emergencies. It is more easily accommodated by a telephone system. The RICA study found no evidence that elderly people considered that the provision of alarms undermined their self esteem or detracted from their valued sense of independence. Instead they provided peace of mind, reassurance and a release from anxiety.

The valuable role of the telephone in keeping in touch with the outside world, especially relatives, is shown in the explanatory study for OFTEL when the whole sample were asked who they contacted. Most calls were made to relatives. What was perhaps equally important was the role of the telephone for other people to talk to this vulnerable group. The majority of the sample either received more calls than they made or claimed to be equally receivers and initiators. There appeared to be an understanding, within families at least, that the cost of phoning long distance would be met by the younger generation.

## PROBLEMS

To look at some of the problems of alarms it is useful to do this against the criteria of what an alarm needs to be.

*Acceptable and understandable.* Research indicates that not all elderly people understand how the alarm operates. They may need to be constantly reminded. Likewise some are reluctant to use it or even to wear it regularly. The RICA study showed that 13% of their sample who had experienced an emergency decided not to use their alarm. In three fifths of these cases this was from feelings of independence or because of lack of confidence about "causing trouble." Steps may need to be taken to overcome the reluctance of some elderly people to use both alarms and telephones. If the reason for the reluctance is cost, for example of the telephone call, some way must be found to solve this problem. One thing which could probably help would be if elderly people could get to know the people who are likely to respond when they are not relatives or friends. In the RICA study nearly one third of clients were visited regularly by alarm service staff and these visits were much appreciated. A large majority (37%) of people who were not visited would have liked visits.

*Technically efficient and easy to operate.* Alarms have become much more sophisticated in recent years and the recent reports by the Consumer's Association shows that most are now safe, free of most technical faults, easy to operate and reliable. However, there is still room for a great deal of improvement in the design and operation of telephones especially for people with specific problems such as the profoundly deaf.

*Accessible following a fall.* The best way an alarm can be accessible following a fall is to ensure that the vulnerable person wears it all the time. This is why pull-cord type alarms (half of which tend to be tied up according to research) are of limited value. In the RICA study nearly a third (30%) of people who had been provided with a portable trigger admitted they did not carry it but left it nearby. In the Staying at Home study no one with the personal alarm had wanted to use the alarm but could not get to it but 9% of the sample overall had had this problem. Overall there is strong evidence of the vulnerability of both those who live alone and the most dependent in the answer to the question about whether they had ever wanted to use it. In the Staying at Home study 12% of those living alone and 16% of the most dependent had experienced this situation with the main cause being a fall or being taken ill. One third of the elderly people had had to wait until someone came round or had to cope on their own.

*Have a guarantee of 24 hour coverage from a control centre and be part of a scheme which has a quick response to emergencies.* Many schemes in UK are run on a very local basis with the control centre in the same town as the people with the alarms. However, partly to share costs, some more centralised schemes have been set up with local authorities and housing associations buying into one system or forming a consortia. Most systems keep a list of relatives and neighbours who will respond to the alarm and ones in the public sector usually have a paid employee such as a peripatetic warden or community nurse as a fall back or, sometimes, as the first person who will respond.

*Part of a system which guarantees access to the person's home.* The problem of access involves ethical questions about the right to privacy. Unless duplicate keys are kept access can become a real problem. In the very sheltered housing study nearly everyone (94%) was allowed to lock their own door, the staff having another key. One quarter of these who were not allowed to lock their own doors were unhappy about this. Most of these said that they wanted more privacy or that it was safer and more secure to lock their own doors. "They just walk in," "They can come in when you're not here." Looking at those in the community the RICA study found that two fifths of the sample had made no arrangements which would allow responders to enter their home if no-one was available to let them in. Twenty-five per cent of the total sample said that the responder would have to break the lock, and, more fatalistically, 15% either just did not know what would happen or admitted that the responder would not be able to get in at all (RICA, 1986, p. 64). In this study responders would have had to go to a neighbour, a warden or get the police to break in. Only a minority (15%) of local authorities had a legal agreement with clients which governed the right of entry.

There are four other problems shown by the research. One is that alarms are *rarely suitable for confused elderly people*, especially those with dementia. The second is that of cost. In the UK alarms are often free of charge if the recipient is a tenant in local authority housing. There is also provision for telephones to be installed under the *Chronically Sick and Disabled Persons Act, 1970*. Some local authorities meet rental charges and some also installation costs but there is not a uniform picture. Some other rebates and concessions are available for people in certain circumstances (e.g., extension bells and watch receivers for the hard of hearing are supplied free of charge to residential customers). Some measure of subsidy may be needed for people whose needs are greatest. DOE advice on personal alarms which can be bought privately says there is need to ensure that the system has reasonable running costs (DOE and Welsh Office, 1988).

The third problem is *lack of information*. In the OFTEL study very few of the people interviewed displayed any interest in special facilities or equipment. One reason was cost but the other was lack of information. Sometimes the information was not available and sometimes it was not very user friendly. There is a need for clearly written, targeted information available in a variety of places. In the UK the obvious place is the doctor's waiting room. One attempt to give more information on alarms is the production of a popular version of the RICA report (Age Concern et al., 1987).

Another issue, which could be considered a problem, is the *lack of interest* by elderly and disabled people in both alarms and telephones. In the Scottish study when asked what they regarded as the three best things about living in sheltered housing only 6% mentioned alarm systems (Clapham and Munro, 1988). In the sheltered housing study in the UK there was little interest in the subject of alarms and over half the tenants said that they did not know that the scheme they were entering would have an alarm system. The initial reaction of many was that though it seemed a good idea it did not have relevance to them personally. In the OFTEL study of telephones there was an almost complete lack of interest in the subject. On one occasion a group of elderly people heard out the interviewer before a planned group discussion and then politely turned back to their bingo. However the RICA study records 63% of elderly people thinking that having an alarm had been a very or fairly good idea.

Other problems have been reported. For example one elderly person took an overdose of aspirins then activated her alarm only to find that the telephone had been cut off because she had not paid the bills. The alarm did not get through although the equipment was working perfectly. This was followed by an agreement between housing authorities and British Telecom to notify one another of the presence of an alarm and any likelihood of disconnection.

## COSTS

The only costings exercise in the UK which includes all the public expenditure costs of keeping a person at home with an alarm is the *Staying at Home* study (Tinker, 1984b). The costs calculated here included the alarm, personal and domiciliary help, doctors visits, housing subsidies and state income benefits. They were updated in the Very Sheltered Housing study (Tinker, 1989b). They show that the staying at home options were the most cost effective. The range of gross costs is shown in Table 1.

## CONCLUSIONS

The main conclusion arising from the research on both alarms and telephones is the importance of providing them as part of a package of community care. Most people who need an alarm are likely to need other services such as help with personal and domestic activities. This points to the need for careful assessment of what is needed taking into account the views of the elderly person and the carer. This fits in very well with the current philosophy of providing packages of care to enable elderly people to remain in the community. Specifically on telephones research shows its key importance for disabled and elderly people and there should be concern about those who do not have the use of one.

Table 1 A comparison of resource costs and transfer payments for a person
of high dependency[1] in hospital, Part III, very sheltered housing,
sheltered housing and staying at home with an innovatory service

| 1986-87 | £ per person per annum | | |
|---|---|---|---|
| | Resource costs [2] | Resource costs and retirement pension or allowance for personal expenses[3] | Resource costs and retirement pension and supplementary pension or allowance for personal expenses[3] |
| Hospital: | | | |
| Acute | 22,014 | 22,417 | 22,417 |
| Geriatric | 19,525 | 19,928 | 19,928 |
| Long-stay | 18,649 | 19,052 | 19,052 |
| | | | |
| Local authority old people's home | 7,844 | 8,247 | 8,247 |
| | | | |
| Very sheltered housing: | | | |
| All | 4,698 | 6,710 | 7,591 |
| 1 bed self-contained | | | |
| New build | 4,842 | 6,854 | 7,735 |
| Rehabilitated | 3,427 | 5,439 | 6,320 |
| | | | |
| Sheltered housing – 1 bed self-contained new-build: | | | |
| Local authority | 4,381 | 6,393 | 7,274 |
| Housing association | 4,359 | 6,371 | 7,252 |
| | | | |
| Innovatory schemes: | | | |
| All | 3,724 | 5,736 | 6,617 |
| Alarms | 3,682 | 5,694 | 6,575 |
| Care | 3,777 | 5,789 | 6,670 |

1,2,3 See Tinker A, An Evaluation of Very Sheltered Housing, HMSO,
London 1989, for details.

## REFERENCES

Age Concern England, Anchor housing association, RICA Calling for help: a guide to emergency alarm systems, Age Concern England et al., Mitcham, Surrey, 1987.

Butler, A and Oldman, C, *Alarm Systems for the Elderly*, Department of Social Policy and Administration, University of Leeds, Leeds, 1981.

Butler, A, Oldman, C and Greve, J, *Sheltered Housing for the Elderly: Policy, Practice and the Consumer*, Allen and Unwin, London, 1983.

Clapham, D and Munro *A Comparison of Sheltered and Amenity Housing for Older People*, Central Research Unit Paper, Scottish Office, Glasgow, 1988.

Consumer's Association, 'Sounding the alarm,' *Which*, Consumers Association, London, November 1988.

Department of Health, *Caring for People: Community Care in the next decade and beyond*, HMSO, London 1989.

Department of the Environment and Welsh Office, *Your home in retirement*, DOE and Welsh Office, London 1988.

Fennell, G, *Anchor's Older People*, Anchor Housing Association, Oxford, 1986.

Fisk, M (ed), *Alarm Systems and Elderly People*, The Planning Exchange, Glasgow, 1989.

Martin, A, White, A and Meltzer, H. *Disabled adults: services, transport and employment*, OPCS, Her Majesty's Stationery Office (HMSO), London, 1989.

McGarry, M. *Community alarm systems for older people*, Age Concern Scotland, Edinburgh, 1985.

OPCS, *General Household Survey 1986*, HMSO, London, 1989.

RICA, *Dispersed alarms: a guide for organisations installing systems*, RICA, London, 1986.

Salvage, *Attitudes of the over 75s to Health and Social Services*, Final report, Research Team for the Care of the Elderly, University of Cardiff, 1986.

Tinker, A. *The Elderly in Modern Society*, Longman, Harlow, 2nd edition, 1984a.

Tinker A. *Staying at Home: Helping elderly people*, HMSO, London 1984b.

Tinker, A. *The Telecommunications Needs of Disabled and Elderly People*. Available from the Library, OFTEL, Atlantic House, Holborn Viaduct, London EC1H 2HQ. price £4.00, 1989a.

Tinker, A. *An Evaluation of Very Sheltered Housing*, HMSO, London, 1989b.

# Community Alarm Systems

## Thomas Breen

### BACKGROUND

In Britain in 1986 there were an estimated 8,495,000 persons aged 65 and over representing some 15.4% of the total population of 55 million. Life expectancy has increased dramatically during this century: from 53 years for those born around 1910 to 75 years for those born now.

There are over 10 million pensioners living in Great Britain, i.e., women over 60 and men over 65 years of age. More than one third of all elderly people and half of those aged over 80 years, live alone. While the vast majority of elderly persons are independent and fit, old age is marked by a gradual deterioration in health and mobility.

Initially Help the Aged was set up to respond to disasters overseas and it was mainly a fundraising charity. Soon, however it began to give grants in the United Kingdom to organizations operating day centres and to other community groups.

Around 1984, demographic trends showed clearly that isolation of elderly people, particularly the over 75's, necessitated the Charity examining ways of dealing with this in a manner which would tie in with the development of community care in the United Kingdom.

Help the Aged established a "Community Alarms Programme" in late 1985 to supply frail, isolated, elderly people with in-home telephone alarm systems. These are special telephones with built-in loudspeakers and microphones that automatically dial a control center when triggered by pressing a button on the telephone unit or on a pendant that is worn by the user (see Photo 1). The control centers are manned 24 hours a day, 365 days a year. In an emergency, help is on hand at the push of a button.

The charity assumes that elderly people in local authority housing will

---

Thomas Breen is affiliated with Help the Aged, England.

*191*

PHOTO 1. Tunstall Telecom's Lifeline 2 Plus unit with integrated telephone and 'Petite' pendant.

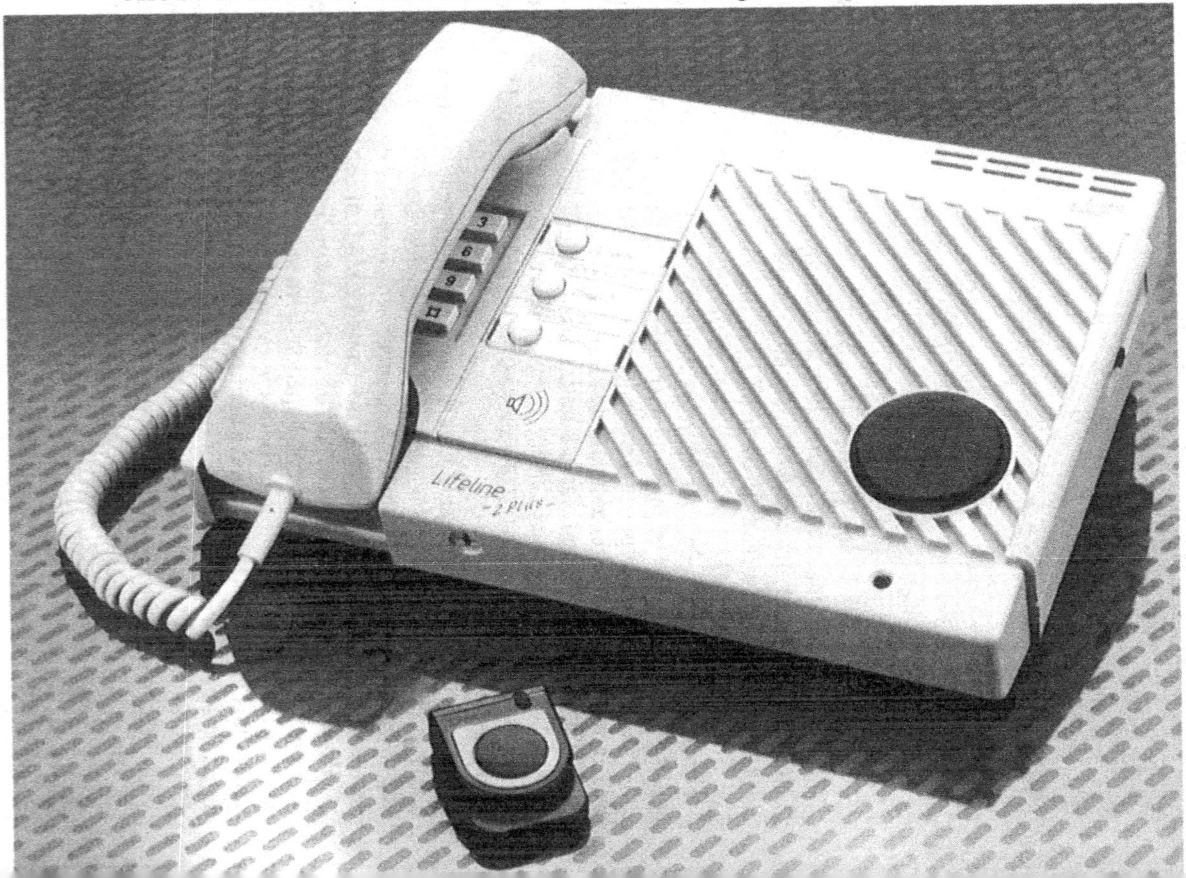

have their alarm needs catered to by the local authority and therefore aim to help needy elderly people in the private sector to remain in their own homes, owned or rented. The Community Alarms Programme is self-financing. Help the Aged act as enablers, facilitators and coordinators, raising funds for purchasing and installation of units plus ongoing monitoring. Funds come mainly from local fund raising for alarms and from cross financing from other agencies. Through this program, Help the Aged have assisted over 11,000 elderly people to obtain monitors since 1985. In 1989 3,648 monitors were installed. In 1990 the projected level of installation was 4,000 monitors.

## FUNDING

We approached this with one rule in mind–all money raised locally would be spent locally on the provision of alarms. To this end we create local groups to operate an appeal in the joint names of the council and Help the Aged. These groups, comprised of well known influential local people, target wealthy individuals and industry and commerce to approach for donations as well as organizing publicity campaigns through local media for raising donations from the general public.

Nationally more and more potential and actual sources have been found by enquiring into a client's background so that, for example, an ex-serviceman or his dependents might qualify for funding via military service benevolent funds, especially the Royal British Legion.

We decided to provide the full purchase cost of the alarm and to pay the full cost of the service for a year, after which the client would be responsible for paying. We would also pay, where necessary, for modifications to a client's telephone line. It is not unknown for us to continue to fund the monitoring cost for two or more years in the event of hardship. When it is no longer needed the control centre operators reallocate the unit to another client. In this way, many of the 10,000 units funded by us will be used possibly four or five times.

## CLIENTS

Although limited in funds it was important to us that our criteria were as broad as possible. They were:

1. Clients must be elderly or elderly disabled (persons of pensionable age).
2. Living alone or sharing a home exclusively with other elderly people, or frequently left alone, or cared for by a resident helper who cannot leave the person, and/or the premises.
3. At risk due to physical condition, e.g., past history of heart condition, strokes, respiratory problems, blackouts, collapses, falls, poor eyesight or blindness, general frailty, poor mobility, anxiety about falling or nervous disability.
4. Able to provide at least one emergency keyholder living nearby.
5. Willing to have an emergency communication system.
6. Able to understand the system and be physically capable of using it.

### *"BUY THEM A PHONE"*

Opponents of technological advances in any field will always find reasons, however spurious, as to why the human race should do things differently. So it has been with alarms. In the face not only of common sense evidence but empirical research carried out by this charity and others, the cry from one or two experts is, "GIVE THEM A TELEPHONE."

Their argument is that what elderly people need is the ability to communicate over distance to friends and relatives, and that in this way their isolation can be alleviated. We believe that alarms have a value incomparable to the lesser cost of an ordinary telephone, and this value lies in the ability to use the instrument remotely, via the radio trigger. If ordinary telephones had this ability, then we would not need a separate alarm and we would not spend our time raising the funds for them.

These opponents point to the contention that as the vast majority of elderly people are quite fit, not prone to falling, all they need is a means for talking to people to ease isolation. This is a narrow view of the process of aging. It is like saying that because I know that I am the safest driver in the world, I do not need a speedometer or brakes. Of course, I may not use the alarm facility for years but one day I may and I will be very thankful that I have ignored the experts and used common sense. Of fatal accidents in the home of people in the age range 65-74, 60% were caused by falls and in the 75+ age group, 86%. Of non-fatal accidents, 60% and 78% were caused by falls for the same age ranges respectively.

### *EQUIPMENT*

Help the Aged telephone alarms are mostly the Lifeline 11 made by Tunstall Telecom, although some Vitalcalls made by Modern Alarms are used. When the elderly people prefer to keep their own telephone, Solo units made by Tunstall are supplied. These are similar to Lifelines but do not have a built in telephone. The main installation requirement is a new style telephone socket and a 13 amp mains socket within twelve feet of each other.

## CONTROL CENTERS

It is estimated that there are 260 control centers run by local authorities servicing around 750,000 people in the United Kingdom. Control centers are manned day and night by full-time employees (see Photo 2). Those monitored are mostly elderly people in sheltered accommodation. Help the Aged have monitoring agreements with, and link their alarms to, 120 control centers who use approved equipment and offer good monitoring services at reasonable prices.

An emergency call initiates two-way communication with the control center. It activates a VDU which displays key data relevant to the person being monitored such as: their name; address; their physical disabilities; name and telephone numbers of people who can be contacted in an emergency; the name of the medical practitioner; friends and relatives.

An emergency call expedites a response from the control center. Either a mobile warden employed by the control center will visit the person, or a neighbor or family member will check up on them. In an emergency, the emergency services can be dispatched.

## CHARGES

The total cost of a monitoring unit is around £220. The control center also charges the customer for the monitoring service; this is usually from 75 pence to £1.50 a week. Help the Aged often raises funds to pay for the alarm and the monitoring service for the first year. After that period, the monitoring service becomes the responsibility of the client, although in cases of hardship the charity may be able to assist with further monitoring bills.

## RESEARCH

As the Community Alarms Programme is rapidly expanding, Help the Aged commissioned a research study to better understand who the main

PHOTO 2. Each Tunstall Lifeline Control Centre gives a 24-hour a day service taking immediate action upon receipt of a call. The colour coded Visual Display Units show details of a caller's situation and health record.

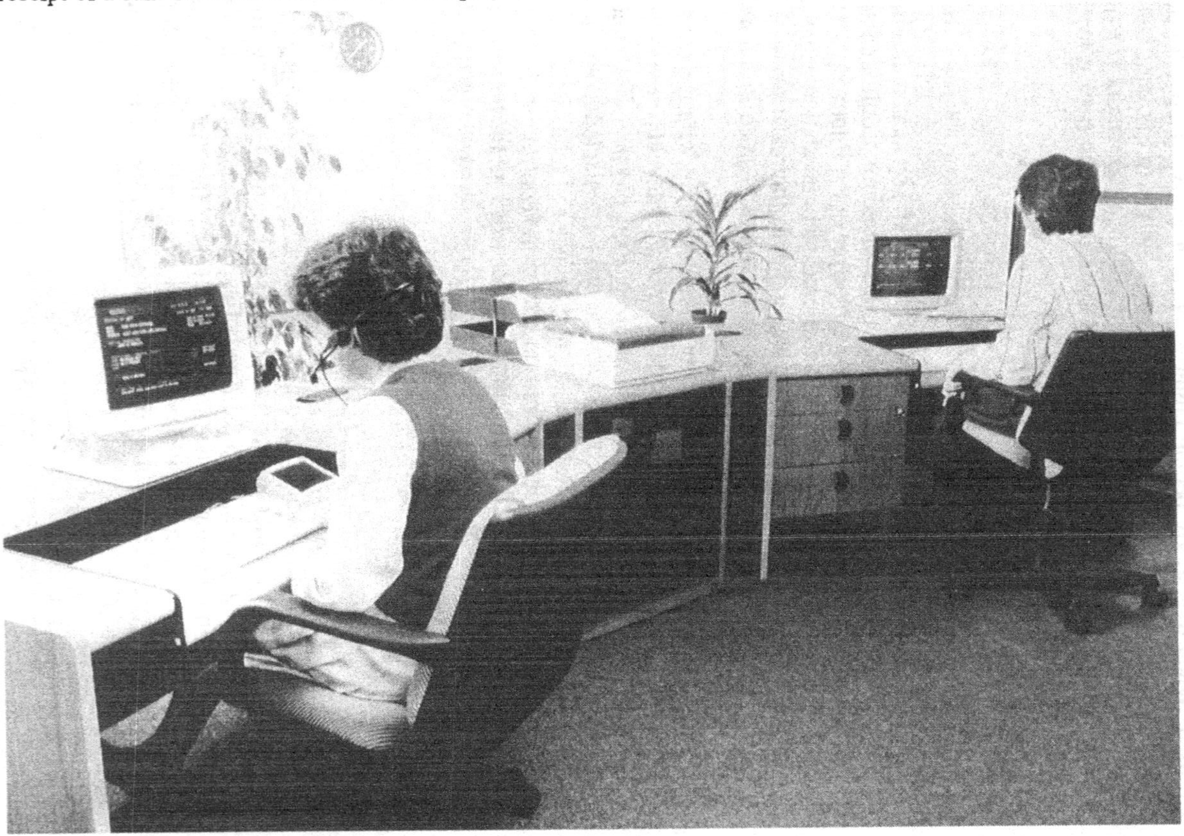

beneficiaries were, how they used the monitoring system, whether there were any technical problems, and identify any further services they could offer to improve the Community Alarms Programme.

The overall objective of this project was to gain a detailed understanding of the recipients of the monitors–both a profile of the types of people using the alarms and the benefits and problems of the alarm to them.

More specifically, the research was designed to: Establish a demographic and lifestyle profile of users; examine the decision process prior to installing a monitor; identifying key influencers and highlighting the key "objections"; identify the barriers to installation; determine recipients attitudes to the monitor once installed, both positives and negatives; examine the day-to-day usage of the monitor including components such as the pendants.

A sample of 350 recipients was randomly drawn for telephone interviews from the total list of 6,000 helped by Help the Aged. Eighty-seven percent were female, average age was upper 70's and all lived in the U.K.

## Profile of Users

Over half of the charity's alarm users own their own homes, and there is a predominance of women.

## Installation of Alarm

a. *Awareness*: There is no clear single source of media information. The alarm is often "introduced" by other people.
b. *Interest*: Initial enquiries for alarms generally occur after a "negative event" (e.g., accident, sickness, or death of a spouse). Falls and fear of falls are one of the main motivators.
c. *Decision*: In many cases the alarm is initially most wanted by other people, not the alarm user. The people most likely to push users into getting an alarm are their children.

Alarm users have an interesting attitude to their children. They say they don't want to bother them; they've got their own lives to lead. They also claim their children do not meddle in their affairs even amongst those people where the children wanted them to have the alarm the most.

These findings indicate the alarm users tend to be people who want to retain their independence and dignity. Given that many of the users are over 80 years old, maybe people leave getting their alarm too late?

d. *Purchase*: Alarms are generally bought by someone else, particularly a charity. Users did contribute to the cost in some cases. This may indicate a passive role in the purchase decision.

### Use of Alarm

Only a third of users are checking their alarms to a level Help the Aged consider adequate, i.e., once a month or more. Most users haven't actually used their alarm in the last month and say they would only use it in a serious emergency. Alarm users like the pendant and wear it frequently, especially the less mobile users. Most think the alarm is good value for money.

### Benefits of the Alarm

The main benefit of the alarm is that it provides reassurance to the users that help is there if it's needed. They commented that they felt safer and not so isolated. Others mentioned it helped them remain independent. The alarm does not appear to affect the level of visitors received by users.

Most users were aware of Help the Aged but are not in contact with them.

### Issues Arising from the Project

The alarm has the desired effect of reassuring recipients and making them feel safer and more confident. However, many do not check their alarms to ensure they are working and use them infrequently. Therefore, it is questionable whether they would be able to use them/obtain the desired response in an emergency. Additionally, 18% of the users are deaf. Would this affect their ability to use the monitor effectively?

These findings may indicate a need for "refresher courses" for those who have had their alarm awhile where they are reminded how to check their alarm. It would also enable someone to reassess the user. Additionally, users may need to be encouraged to use the alarm in more non-life threatening situations to increase the frequency of use.

## WHAT OF THE FUTURE?

The elements that brought us into this campaign are not going to go away tomorrow. They are:

- Growing numbers of elderly people
- Growing isolation in later years
- Community care to expand in the United Kingdom
- Care charges for individuals to become more frequent
- Technology development
- Community alarms as a part of a broad care package for elderly people.

The one element which captures our imagination and which allows a vision of the future, is the progress in the development of the technology. Already we know of pilot projects to test equipment which can monitor patients' vital signs–a telephone style instrument. Heart beat, pulse rate and blood pressure can be monitored over the telephone network. The implications for the present concept of hospitals' outpatient services are enormous.

Some countries have already made great strides in using the public service telephone network for home shopping, banking and other aspects of daily life. All of these advances are to be welcomed, for in opposing them we merely seek to hold back the ocean of progress. Above all is the need for our independent 'watch' over the quality of provision, not leaving elderly people to have the potential pitfalls of an explosion of market forces.

# UNITED STATES

# Personal Response Systems
# in the United States

### Christina Montgomery

## *INTRODUCTION*

This paper will be divided into five distinct sections; historical overview, analysis of the current Personal Response Systems (PRS) market,
benefits of PRS, barriers to usage and future trends. These five sections,
when viewed in totality, should provide a thorough understanding of PRS
in the United States through its inception, the current trends and barriers to
growth and the future of this rapidly expanding industry.

The section on the history of PRS in the United States will be an
overview of Lifeline Systems, Inc. the primary developer of PRS in the
U.S. and Canada. Currently Lifeline Systems commands 65 to 70% of the
sold market with over 250,000 people utilizing the Lifeline service
throughout the U.S. and Canada. There will be a discussion of growth
through the 80s with the entrance of other companies into the PRS market
in the U.S.

The analysis of the current PRS market will focus on demographic
information on current users, variances in technology and the structure and

---

Christina Montgomery is Corporate Sales Manager, New Business Development Lifeline Systems, Inc.

*201*

delivery of the service. This section will also address the current cost of the equipment and monitoring charges as well as who pays usually for the service.

The section on the benefits of PRS will be divided into two distinct segments; benefits to the user, their family and caregivers and benefits to the health care system with implications regarding the need to expand third party reimbursement for the service.

Understanding the barriers to usage is critical if we are to develop successful strategies to overcome these barriers in the 90s and bring this service to all those who need it and can benefit from it. This section will focus primarily on the research undertaken by Lifeline Systems, Inc. to better understand how to deliver PRS to the expanding market of both the elderly and the medically vulnerable as well as those non-elderly individuals who may want PRS for a variety of reasons other than medical.

Future developments in PRS will focus on both system changes and technological advances. System changes will primarily involve changes in the health care delivery system with respect to access and cost; especially as the U.S. health care system attempts to cope with the growing number of people over the age of 65. Technological advances will involve changes that will remove barriers to usage as well as advances that will expand PRS to other market segments such as the physically challenged and chronically ill, non-elderly.

The primary objective of this paper is to provide a thorough overview of PRS in the U.S. and to stimulate questions and dialogue regarding the changes required to bring PRS to more people who need and want it in the 90s and on into the 21st century.

## HISTORICAL OVERVIEW

Personal Response Systems in the U.S. have a relatively brief history, approximately sixteen years. However, what it lacks in longevity is more than made up for in growth, now serving over 350,000 individuals in all fifty states and in Canada. The concept of PRS was first developed by Dr. Andrew Dibner at Duke University in 1973. A three year study supported by a grant from the National Center for Health Services Research in 1975 and utilizing Lifeline equipment and response protocols resulted in four general findings (Sherwood & Morris, 1980).

1. INDEPENDENT LIVING
   Lifeline users felt more comfortable about living alone and more confident about continuing to live independently.

2. DAYS OF NURSING HOME CARE
For each day spent in a nursing home by Lifeline users, nonusers required 13 days.

3. COST/BENEFIT
For users of Lifeline who were severely functionally disabled and not socially isolated each $1.00 of Lifeline services produced a net savings of $7.19 in total long-term care costs due to reduced use of institutional and community care.

4. RATE OF EMERGENCIES
The emergency rate for the frail population was approximately 1/2 per user per year, or an average of 1 each week for every 100 users. 73% of these emergencies were health related and 27% were environmental.

The results of this study gave a clear signal that the development of Lifeline or similar Personal Response Systems was justified both from a cost/benefit perspective and from the qualitative perspective of the user. With this knowledge Lifeline Systems, Inc. began to market its services in 1979 (see Photo 1).

Lifeline trained a field sales force to sell the service through hospitals and other health care facilities. These health care facilities established Response Centers, usually in their emergency rooms staffed 24 hours per day, and rented the Lifeline equipment to a user, living alone and/or at risk, for a monthly fee; approximately $10-12.00 per month. During the early 80s many hospitals marketed the Lifeline service to the frail elderly who lived alone primarily as a community service; thus bringing to the hospital a positive community image and valuable public relations. Even though research such as the Ruchlin and Morris study, 1981, focused on the positive cost/benefit analysis of the Lifeline service most health care facilities did not focus on the critical factors of cost containment through the use of PRS until the mid 80s.

By the mid 80s Lifeline had introduced a voice product to accompany the non-voice unit and had placed over 100,000 people on the service. New companies offering PRS had entered the market thus bringing to the consumer a wide variance in the type of products and services available. Companies that were in the security and alarm business began to offer PRS as an additional service. Small "mom and pop" companies also began to emerge, selling equipment purchased through manufacturers of automatic dialers and alarm devices. Three distinct trends developed in the last half of the 80s:

1. Centralized toll-free monitoring using 800 telephone lines began a steady growth pattern with all PRS companies.
2. Direct to consumer businesses offering PRS began to expand by offering franchises and/or distributorships and augmenting sales with intensive media advertising.
3. Two-way voice communication equipment became "state of the art" as the way to meet the needs of an expanding and diverse market as well as to reduce the number of false alarms requiring intervention.

PHOTO 1. A Lifeline 5000 communicator in the home.

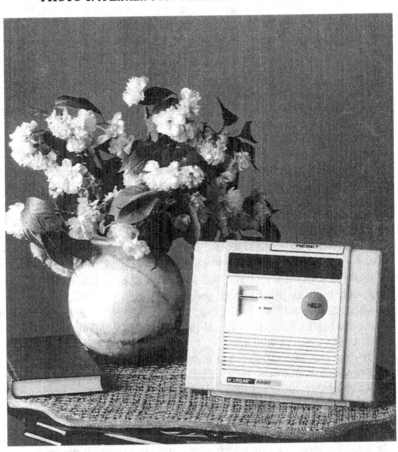

Also during the mid 80s a major shift in the structure of the government subsidized health care payment system took place. Traditionally U.S. health care has been a "fee for service" type system with payments limited only by what had been viewed as "reasonable and customary" on the part of the provider of service, usually a physician. With rising health care costs that appeared to be spiraling out of control, the U.S. government attempted to apply some measure of control with a prospective payment system under Medicare, the health care program for those over age 65. This system installed a classification system called DRGs, Diagnostic Related Groups. Based on a DRG classification for a patient, the hospital was allotted a fixed dollar amount and a fixed length of stay. Hospitals were forced to provide quality care within a predetermined framework, a specific fixed dollar amount and a specific length of stay.

This fundamental change in the infrastructure of the U.S. health care system had and will continue to have a very strong effect on the PRS industry. Due to the fact that Lifeline has the lion's share of the sold PRS market and that this market is predominately through hospitals, it became critical that hospital-based Lifeline programs restructure themselves to become financially self-sufficient. Although still an excellent community service, PRS are even more compelling when viewed as a mechanism that can assist in reducing length of hospital stay, avoiding inappropriate admissions and providing a "bonded" patient base to which a hospital can market other health care services in what is an extremely competitive marketplace. Since PRS in the U.S. is a private pay service primarily offered through hospitals and not a public service it is critical to keep the hospital based PRS programs financially healthy.

PRS companies selling in the health care market have had to restructure their products and services to meet the changes delineated above. Reducing the labor intensity of running a PRS program and enhancing the products to meet the needs of new market segments were keys to success in the late 80s and will also be key to continued industry vitality in the 90s.

Lifeline's development of a self-installable unit and LifeTrac, a software package to automate call response have been successful attempts at reducing labor intensity. The use of toll-free centralized monitoring as opposed to on-site monitoring also reduces labor costs as well as liability concerns. Lifeline's introduction of the Access Package for the physically challenged have expanded the accessibility of Lifeline to this group of individuals who truly need it to live independently. Special adaptive switches can modify the Personal Call Button for use by an individual who does not have the manual ability to press it. The Access Package allows for ease of phone answering by use of the adaptive switch and also includes a smoke alarm which is integrated into the Response System. The Access Package has allowed hospitals to expand their PRS programs to the physically challenged, allowing a significant number of people to live independently and with dignity. The much hoped for by-product of the larger hospital based PRS program is that it can become financially self sufficient and thus serve all those who need and want the service, including the indigent client.

## PRS INDUSTRY OVERVIEW–CURRENT SITUATION

In 1989 Lifeline placed its 200,000th unit and also celebrated its 15th anniversary. Currently in the U.S. there are approximately 30 plus companies offering Personal Response Systems with almost the total market share controlled by six to seven companies. As a result over 350,000 people now live more independently and with greater dignity.

This section of the paper will be a "snapshot" of the current state of the PRS industry in the United States. The focus will be two pronged; a demographic analysis of the users of PRS and an analysis of the delivery of the Personal Response Service to the user, reviewing how the services are monitored, cost, types of equipment and who pays for the service.

### Demographic Analysis

Although exact figures are not available industry-wide, it is estimated that well over 350,000 people are utilizing PRS in the U.S. Research shows that the great majority of these users are elderly, over the age of 70. A survey of Lifeline Program Managers in 1989 found the average user age to be 74 while an analysis of users subscribing to Lifeline Central, Lifeline Systems' toll-free central monitoring service, found the average age to be 84 (Patel, 1989). Another study undertaken by Lifeline Systems found that of 1,754 users responding to a survey 39% were between 76-85 years with 28% in the 85+ group (Lifeline Systems, Inc., 1989).

Women are the primary users of PRS constituting 76% in the Lifeline Program Manager survey and over 80% in previously mentioned Lifeline survey of 1,754 users (see Photo 2). Many of these women are widowed and living alone (Patel, 1989).

When reviewing the medical history of current PRS users, most of them suffer from one or more chronic illnesses. When Lifeline Program Managers were asked to list the four most common chronic illnesses of their users

PHOTO 2. Woman wearing Lifeline portable help button.

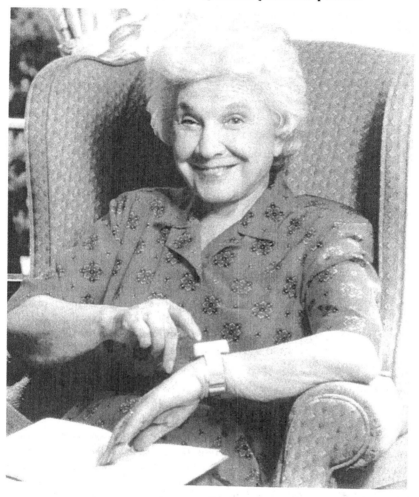

they list cardiac, arthritis, diabetes and stroke. The Lifeline Central survey found agreement with the above survey results and also found hypertension and emphysema/chronic obstructive lung disease common to many subscribers (Lifeline, 1989).

Call emergencies often reflect a correlation with these chronic illnesses;

with falls, cardiovascular and respiratory related emergency calls predominating. In a Lifeline Central survey of approximately 950 users over six months, there were a total of 228 incidents with the most frequent four types of incidents logged as follows:

| TYPE OF EMERGENCY | NUMBER LOGGED |
|---|---|
| 1. Falls | 109 |
| 2. Not Well | 24 |
| 3. Difficulty Breathing | 16 |
| 4. Chest Pain | 15 |

The average length of stay on PRS is not well documented industry wide. However, a recent survey by Dr. Dibner found it to be 10.5 months with most users terminating due to death or the need for a higher level of care such nursing home placement (Dibner, 1990).

When users are asked who referred them to a PRS, most often the answer is a friend or the hospital. A Lifeline User's Survey found that a hospital, a friend or a relative are the three top referral sources voiced by the user. Often in the hospital setting a social worker or discharge planner will be the key staff person to recommend a PRS to a patient. Family members, especially the potential user's child, are usually the most influential in getting them to use a PRS (Patel, 1989).

### Equipment and Delivery of Service

A Personal Response System consists of three components: a portable transmitter worn by the user; a communicator which is attached to the user's telephone; and a response center to receive the calls from the user's home. Primarily the service is delivered to the user in two ways: through a health care facility for a monthly fee or through companies that sell the equipment directly to the end-user through the use of a direct sales force and media advertising. Monitoring is undertaken either by the hospital itself or through centralized toll free contract monitoring by the company selling the equipment. Historically the monitoring has been community based through hospitals which developed their own PRS programs. However, over the past few years there has developed a shift to centralized monitoring to accommodate the growing number of users and the health care industry's staffing problems and financial concerns.

The in-home equipment generally costs between $500 to 800; however, some direct to consumer companies charge between $1700 and $2,000.

Installation and training fees also vary across the industry from $30 to $175. Monitoring costs range from $35 to $45 per month and often includes the rental of the equipment. Some hospital-based programs charge $20 or less per month, subsidizing their PRS with community raised funds and grants and utilizing volunteers to manage the program (Dibner, 1990).

The end user usually pays for the PRS although in some instances a relative will help with the monthly charges. Hospital-based PRS have often developed sponsorships with church and civic groups as well as social service agencies.

Formal third-party coverage is limited in the PRS industry at the present time. Private insurance companies occasionally pay for PRS on a case-by-case basis, especially with a written recommendation from the user's physician. Nineteen states include PRS under their Medicaid Home and Community Support Based Services Waiver Programs covering approximately 8,000 people, and Massachusetts is the only state that covers PRS under its Medicaid DME (Durable Medical Equipment) regulations.

The state of New York will soon offer PRS to qualifying clients under their Personal Care Program which should make over 20,000 clients eligible for PRS coverage. In some cases Area Agencies on Aging have made funds available for hospital-based PRS to purchase equipment for indigent clients. In many cases a Medicaid client will be placed on a waiting list if third party support to cover the monthly fees is not available. Even with the third party coverage mechanisms listed above and the efforts of hospital-based PRS programs to assist with sponsorship and sliding scale fee structures there are many people who need a Personal Response System and cannot obtain it due to lack of funds.

## BENEFITS OF PERSONAL RESPONSE SYSTEMS

The benefits of a PRS can be easily divided into three categories:

1. Benefits to the user.
2. Benefits to the caregiver.
3. Benefits to the health care system.

The benefits to the user are both psychosocial and financial in regard to medical care. Numerous studies have shown that individuals using PRS state they have a heightened feeling of security and peace of mind. In the initial study of Lifeline by Sherwood and Morris (1980) Lifeline users "felt more comfortable about living alone and were more confident about continuing to live independently." Recently, Lifeline Systems completed a user survey (Patel, 1989) and found that when users were asked, "What is the number one benefit of Lifeline to you?", users replied:

1. Quick help if needed          42% of the responses
2. Security                      24% of the responses
3. Peace of mind                 13% of the responses

During a Lifeline Central survey in 1989 many users expressed in their own words why the Lifeline service was so beneficial to them. Following are some direct quotations from Lifeline users:

"I have the gift of independence . . . its a wonderful thing." "I fell in my garage once *without* Lifeline and laid there for many hours." "I had a stroke and I want to live alone."

These comments reinforce the fact that most people who opt for a PRS do so for security and peace of mind. They repeatedly comment on that fact that they feel more security with the knowledge that they can get assistance very quickly, even if they cannot get to a telephone. For many users a PRS is the difference between remaining independent in their own home or having to have someone live with them to provide custodial care or be placed in a nursing home. As one Lifeline user stated when asked why she obtained a Lifeline unit, "Because my kids wanted someone to move in."

Often the family of a potential PRS user is instrumental in getting them to use the system. In many cases this is because the family member has some level of caregiving responsibility for their elderly relative. Surveys such as the one by Travelers Corporation, an insurance company in Hartford, Connecticut, and AARP, found that one out of five Traveler's employees over age 30 devoted an average of 10.2 hours per week to caring for an elderly parent; 8% spent 35 hours or more per week providing care to a parent (AARP & Travelers, 1989). Employees concerned with caring for an elderly family member are often not focused on their work; they are distracted and less productive, spend excessive time on the phone checking on the family member and often miss work due to demanding caregiver needs. In some cases caregivers have left the work environment permanently to provide full-time care to an elderly parent or relative.

The utilization of a PRS can, in many instances, relieve the anxiety the caregiver experiences when they cannot physically be with their elderly parent or family member. As one Lifeline user commented, "I think it's terrific . . . it takes a lot of worry off my family." In addition, the cost of a PRS at approximately a dollar a day is much less than live-in supervised care. In the current economic environment over half of the U.S. women work outside the home–most do so out of necessity. Women, society's traditional caregivers, are often sandwiched between meeting the demands of their jobs and meeting the caregiving demands of their elderly family members. They cannot afford to quit work nor can many families afford the cost of live-in care. A PRS can provide both a financial benefit as well as a psychosocial benefit to families that today provide approximately 80% of the care that the elderly receive in the United States. The utilization of PRS as an eldercare service will increase dramatically in the 90s.

The financial benefits of PRS have been documented for well over a decade, mainly through research conducted on the Lifeline Systems, Inc. model of equipment and response protocol. In Sherwood and Morris' 1980 study of elderly tenants in the Boston and Cambridge, Massachusetts Housing Authority, three separate groups were designated depending on the degree of physical frailty and social isolation. A total sample of 551 persons were chosen and randomly designated as either Experimental (were offered Lifeline) and Controls (were not offered Lifeline). At the end of the three year study a cost/benefit analysis was completed on the two targeted matched samples resulting in a 7.19 benefit/cost ratio which indicates that for every one dollar spent on Lifeline there was a resulting savings of $7.19. Cost savings were also found regarding delay of nursing home placement in the Sherwood study; for every one day of nursing placement for the Experimentals, the Controls required 13 days.

Dibner and Stafford (1984) completed a national survey of Lifeline Programs. Surveys were returned by 335 Lifeline Program Managers in 47 states, a response rate of 49%, with data collected on 9,262 Lifeline users. Findings show that 7% of the users spent less time in acute care hospitals because of having a Lifeline unit in their home. In addition, 16% of the users reported a delay in long-term care placement as a result of the Lifeline service. When asked how many hospital days were saved due to the Lifeline service, respondents reported that in 87% of the cases the user's hospital stay was shortened from one to seven days.

Regarding previous discussions on the U.S. health care's prospective payment system which limits payment and length of stay, there are compelling financial benefits for hospital with a PRS that can assist in reducing the length of stay when appropriate. The typical cost of a day in a U. S. hospital is, at a minimum, $539 per day. If we refer to the Stafford and Dibner study, 7% (679) users spent less time hospitalized and 87% of that group (591 users) had their length of stay shortened by at least one day, the potential net savings is $318,549.

The study by Koch (1984) found that the utilization of a PRS assisted with discharge planning. Koch reported reduced hospital admissions for users of PRS as well as a 26% reduction in length of hospital stay.

Dibner (1985) replicated the Koch's retrospective longitudinal study with 70 Lifeline users associated with four Boston hospitals. User's medical records were compared the year following installation of a Lifeline unit to the three years prior to installation. Variables compared were hospital admissions, inpatient days and emergency room visits over this four year period. Findings, even when statistically adjusting for a general trend toward decreased hospital use, reflected a 26.4% decrease in admissions, a 23.2% decrease in length of stay and a 6.5% decrease in emergency room visits during the year after Lifeline was installed.

In addition to reducing length of stay through early discharge, a PRS system can assist the user in obtaining assistance early in a medical emergency, thus preventing more complicated medical intervention and an extended length of stay. A PRS can also assist in providing the appropriate level of medical intervention and in some cases avoid inappropriate admissions and emergency room visits.

Cain (1987) utilized a similar retrospective analysis as the Dibner and Koch studies and found that with 48 PRS users, admissions to a hospital decreased by 48.4% and inpatient hospital days decreased by 69.3%. In an on-going study through the Veteran's Administration (Freedman, 1989) an interim report on 60 users supports the findings of Dibner, Koch, and Cain.

In 1987 the State of New York undertook two separate studies which focused on the cost benefits of utilizing a PRS to reduce the amount of care given to PRS users by Personal Care Attendants (Coordinated Care Management Corporation). One study completed by the New York City Human Resources Administration Medical Assistance Program (1988) found that on the average, 172 PRS users required 91.2 fewer hours of Personal Care each month; a savings of $565 per client per month. The study by Coordinated Care Management Corporation of Buffalo, New York found that PRS users required 144 fewer hours of Personal Care at a savings of $956 per client per month.

In reviewing the research on PRS over the past decade there is clear evidence of the cost benefits to the U.S. health care system in general with respect to five areas:

1. Decreased days in a long-term care setting.
2. Decreased hospital admissions.

3. Decreased length of hospital stay.
4. Decreased use of more expensive health care delivery systems such as Personal Care Attendants.
5. Decreased Emergency Room visits.


Currently, the typical PRS user is elderly (over 70), female, widowed and living alone. Many suffer from one or more medical problems which are chronic in nature and require frequent interaction with the health care delivery system. These individuals are hospitalized nearly twice as often as the younger population; 39.5% of the elderly (65+) population require hospitalization annually and stay an average of 8.7 days as opposed to 7.2 days as a national average (AARP, 1987). The average cost of a day in the hospital is conservatively estimated to be $539 and all indications are that this figure will continue to escalate over the next decade.

The struggle for U.S. hospitals is to maintain financial viability by continuing to admit patients when appropriate for treatment, discharge as soon as appropriate medically, and to provide quality care, whenever possible, at a lesser level which is more cost effective. If health care can be provided adequately outside the hospital through outpatient or ambulatory care centers or in the clients home, the cost is significantly decreased. Personal Response Systems have proven that clients can be cared for in the home and still receive appropriate health care assistance when necessary.

A PRS allows intervention and assessment to take place early in an emergency, thus avoiding an escalation of the medical problem and a higher level of health care delivery–admission to a hospital. This is not to say that a PRS cannot augment hospital admissions by expanding market share. Lifeline Systems' research with hospital-based Lifeline Programs have found that Lifeline users bond with a hospital and that when admission is necessary and appropriate, the user will choose the hospital offering the Lifeline service because of the Lifeline connection. In a similar vein, Lifeline users will also utilize outpatient services based on the facility that provided their Lifeline unit. These factors, plus the ability to affect early discharge, are all beneficial to a hospital.

Lifeline's research with their hospital-based programs has estimated the indirect revenue benefits for a Lifeline program based on its ability to attract and retain patients, increase utilization of outpatient services and assist with appropriate early discharge. The following is an overview of the indirect revenue benefits for a 500 unit hospital-based Lifeline program (Lifeline, 1989).

*Indirect Revenue Benefits:*
*500 Unit Hospital-Based Lifeline Program*

Attracting and Retaining Patients:

| | |
|---|---:|
| 1. Number of Lifeline users: | 500 |
| 2. Thirty-nine point five per cent of users requiring hospitalization: | 198 |
| 3. Number that would use the facility even if Lifeline were not available: | 158 |
| 4. Number that would use the facility because of the Lifeline connection: | 40 |
| 5. Average length of stay (days): | 8.7 |
| 6. Number of patient days due to Lifeline connection: | 348 |
| 7. Average value of one day of hospitalization: | $539 |
| 8. Indirect revenue benefits of Lifeline in attracting patients: | $187,572 |

*Enhancing Utilization of Outpatient Services*

| | |
|---|---:|
| 1. Number of Lifeline users: | 500 |
| 2. Number of outpatient services visits (1.2 times per year/user): | 600 |
| 3. Number that would use the facility even if Lifeline were not available: | 480 |
| 4. Number that would use the facility because of the Lifeline connection: | 120 |
| 5. Average value of outpatient service visit: | $150 |
| 6. Indirect revenue benefit of Lifeline in enhancing outpatient usage: | $18,000 |

*Cost Effective Discharge Planning*

| | |
|---|---:|
| 1. Number of hospital beds at the facility: | 200 |
| 2. Typical bed occupancy (68%): | 136 |
| 3. Average Length of stay: | 7.2 days |
| 4. Average Number of discharges per week: | 132 |
| 5. Three of every 100 patients discharged can be discharged one day earlier with Lifeline (patients per week): | 4 |

6. Number of patients discharged one day early
   per year: 208
7. Average value of one day of hospitalization: $539
8. Indirect revenue benefit of Lifeline through
   early discharge: $112,112

When totalled, the yearly indirect revenue benefits for the hospital are estimated to be $317,648. The hospital has established a cost-effective health care service which is financially self-sustaining. It receives appropriate admissions and outpatient services it would otherwise lose to another facility and it has a service that can assist with early discharge.

In today's health care market hospitals can no longer run programs which cannot pay for themselves. Programs and services are closely scrutinized with regard to their cost as well as their match to the goals and objectives of the facility. A Personal Response System offers a hospital the ability to generate positive public relations by allowing their users to live independently and with peace of mind while creating a cost-effective health care delivery system that allows for early intervention and assessment for an appropriate level of care and early discharge when possible. In addition, by expanding the program beyond the elderly to other groups such as the physically challenged and the non-elderly chronically ill the hospital enhances its opportunity to expand market share while maintaining financial viability. Since the majority of PRS users are serviced through hospitals it is critical to keep these programs financially healthy. Hospital-based PRS programs that are actively growing will remain financially sound and will be able to provide the service to all who need it, regardless of their ability to pay.

## BARRIERS TO USAGE

Unfortunately, even when a Personal Response System is made available there are still several distinct barriers keeping people from utilizing the service. During 1989 Lifeline Systems, Inc. compiled research from nine separate sources with regard to barriers to the usage of a Personal Response product (Patel, 1989).

These sources included surveys of Lifeline Program Managers, Lifeline users, Lifeline Sales Representatives, physicians as well as an analysis of advertising campaigns run by Lifeline. Both managers of Lifeline Programs as well as users of the service voiced similar comments when asked why a potential user might not accept the service. When Lifeline Managers were asked, "What do you see as the primary reasons why a potential user may not choose the system," the four top answers ranked by frequency of mention were:

1. Denial of System Need.
2. Fixed Income/Cost of System.
3. Loss of Independence with System.
4. Will not admit to being old or frail.

When users themselves were surveyed their responses were strikingly similar. When asked to mark an X next to those reasons listed which strongly explained why people who could benefit from Lifeline do not get it, users mentioned:

1. Denial That Service is Needed  (42%).
2. Cannot Afford the System  (34%).
3. They will not admit to becoming older and needing help  (18%).

Users were then asked to add any other reason they wanted that was not listed previously to describe why a potential user would not accept the service. Two answers were most frequent; "unaware service exists" and "do not know procedure of how to obtain." Lastly, current users were asked if they had any hesitation about obtaining Lifeline for themselves; the top two "yes" answers involved: (1) Cost/Extra expense/felt I couldn't afford; and (2) Felt I didn't need it/too proud.

Overall the two major barriers are denial of need and perceived high cost. With regard to the denial of need, many elderly people do not perceive a Personal Response System as relating to their lifestyle. They do not respond positively to technology that singles them out as being old or medically vulnerable. In an article, "Why Seniors Don't Use Technology" (Bowe, 1988) points to seniors resisting products that are symbols of their aging even when the product could make life easier. They feel these products call attention to the fact they are aging and may require special assistance. Also research shows that elderly people see themselves much younger than they actually are; sometimes as much as 10 to 15 years younger. In a survey by Moschis (1989) it was found that seniors generally perceive themselves as feeling and looking younger than their actual age. Seniors in this survey also voiced that they had interests similar to people under the age of sixty and tended to do most things as though they were under the age of sixty. Moschis concluded that the older a person is chronologically the younger they perceive themselves.

These attitudes are related to the potential user's refusal to accept a

Personal Response System even when they could benefit from it. In their view they are still perceiving themselves as capable, independent and younger than they really are. A Personal Response System singles them out from younger people and labels them as vulnerable, not capable of living without assistance. As Personal Response System companies expand the service to other market segments such as the physically challenged, latch key children, single women living alone, and non-elderly population groups who are at risk the elderly may begin to accept that PRS are not just for the elderly but are for all ages.

The cost of the service was also viewed as a barrier. However, there are two ways to view cost as a barrier to usage; actual and perceived. When some seniors state that the cost is too much for the service it is related to their perceived need for the service and not to their actual ability to pay for the service. Here again the senior does not perceive that the product has worth due to the fact that they do not feel they *need* it.

There are, however, many elderly in this country that are on fixed incomes. In 1987 the AARP's Profile of Older Americans stated that 3.5 million elderly persons were below the poverty line ($6,630 for an older couple household and $5,255 for an older individual living alone). Another 2.3 million were classified as being "near poor." Older women had a higher poverty rate at 15% than older men (8%), while older persons living alone or with non-relatives were more likely to experience poverty (25%) than older people living with their families (6%). In comparing race, 31% of elderly Blacks are classified as poor with 23% of elderly Hispanics and 11% of elderly Whites. For these elderly Americans it is not so much a perceived inability to afford the service but an economic fact.

These people, if they need the service and cannot find some type of third party coverage, will not receive it. They are often put on a waiting list if they cannot pay. As discussed earlier in this paper, third party coverage is infrequent, whether through Medicaid or the private sponsorship of civic and community groups. Historically, Personal Response System users have been elderly women living alone. It is this group that has the highest poverty rates as reflected in the AARP survey and in the next decade this group will continue to expand. By the year 2000 persons 65 and older will represent 13% of the U.S. population and by 2030 there will be an estimated 65 million older people. For many Americans the inability to pay for a Personal Response unit is a fact; it is a "luxury" they cannot afford even when they need it and when its use would deter costlier health care intervention.

The research on barriers to usage by Lifeline Systems, Inc. found an additional, secondary barrier–lack of awareness. Although not mentioned with the frequency of the previously discussed barriers, it was mentioned in six of the nine studies undertaken. When physicians were interviewed regarding the Lifeline service most were not resistant to recommending it, they were simple not aware of the service. Often users stated that they were not only unaware of the existence of Personal Response Systems but they also did not know how to go about obtaining one. In follow-up to a Lifeline advertising campaign, two out of every five potential users and/or caregivers knew of the concept of PRS but could not name any companies that provided the service. With PRS being available nationwide through a variety of companies and through over 2400 hospitals there is still strong evidence that the level of awareness regarding this service is low.

In summation, barriers to usage most often involve the denial of need and high cost (perceived or actual) on the part of the potential user. A secondary barrier is lack of awareness by both the potential user as well as the caregiver.

## FUTURE TRENDS

This final section will be divided into two segments; first, a brief discussion of several important trends that will dramatically impinge on the infrastructure of the U.S. health care system; and second, an overview of future trends in the PRS industry. This latter segment will focus on the overall objective of delivering the PRS to as many individuals as possible who can use the service. This will entail the development of products and services as well as marketing approaches that will remove the barriers to usage.

As we look forward into the 90s there are a number of trends that will effect the delivery and the cost of health care in the United States. In 1986 the number of persons 65+ was approximately 29.2 million, 12.1% of the total population. By the year 2000 this number will increase to 34.9 million (13.0%). The 55-64 age group is expected to grow by a rate of 77% between 1987 and 2015. The "baby boomers" born after World War II will reach age 65 between 2010 and 2030 with 64.6 million people 65+ in 2030, 21.1% of the total population (AARP, 1987).

People are living much longer today. A child born in 1986 in the U.S. will have a life expectancy of about 74.9 years, approximately 28 years longer than a child born in 1900. Medical technology and treatment have contributed to a longer life span. Today people are living longer with chronic health conditions that would not have been survivable twenty years ago (AARP, 1987).

In 1984 the 65+ population accounted for 31% of the total health care dollars spent in the U.S. This was estimated to be approximately $120 billion, of which 45% was hospital based expenditures for care of the 65+ age group (AARP, 1987). As the U.S. population continues to age over the next three decades the current health care delivery system will be hard pressed to meet their needs.

Other problems face the health care industry today. There is a critical shortage of long-term care beds in this country. Many people who truly require nursing home care cannot find a bed and are placed on waiting lists. As the population ages this shortage will take on even more critical proportions.

Most U.S. families are either dual income or single working woman, head of household. This impacts the ability of the family to provide care to an aging parent as was the case in the past. In addition, many elderly do not live with family members but live alone; about 30% of non-institutionalized elderly live alone and this figure is increasing faster than the elderly population in general.

The AIDS crisis has and will continue to place demands on the health care delivery system. Hospital-based treatment for AIDS is expensive and prolonged as with any chronic illness. With the expected increases in AIDS over the next decade, the health care system will have to look for alternatives to inpatient care.

Lastly, third party coverage is insufficient to cover the health care cost of many Americans. If not privately insured through an employee benefits plan, many Americans cannot afford to buy insurance but have too much income to be eligible for Medicaid. The AARP Profile of Older Americans found that third party coverage, whether it be Medicare, Medicaid or other government programs, covered approximately two thirds of the health care expenditure for elderly people and only about one third for persons under age 65 in 1984.

All these factors add up to a crisis in American health care delivery over the next three decades. As the health care industry looks to reduce its delivery costs more services will be developed outside the traditional institutional settings. Home health care and social HMOs will continue to grow providing both medical and social care in a more cost effective manner. Nursing homes are developing services for potential residents including delivery of meals and home care, an extension of the concept "nursing home without walls." The senior housing market is integrating many "assisted living" concepts into their facilities with the realization that their current residents will be aging in place and requiring higher levels of care. Corporations are evaluating eldercare and other employee benefits such as long-term care insurance for their retirees, aging work force and for their employee caregivers. As solutions are developed both in the public and private section to alleviate this crisis the PRS industry has a unique opportunity to assist in reducing the costs of health care delivery by allowing people to live independently in their own homes.

In order to meet the opportunity to bring a Personal Response System to as many people as possible there are three challenges the industry will have to overcome in the 90s:

1. Remove the barriers to usage.
2. Expand the service to all population groups, regardless of age, who need it.
3. Create an industry wide code of ethics–quality of product and service.

As previously discussed, the barriers to PRS usage involve denial of need, cost of product, (both perceived and actual) and lack of willingness to admit to being old, frail or handicapped. The industry will need to focus on increased product acceptability in the 90s. This will come through the development of products and services that can be utilized by not only the elderly but the non-elderly as well; products and services that can be integrated into the lifestyles of seniors as well as younger people. Only then will the elderly be willing to accept PRS. As stated earlier in the Barriers section, elderly persons do not accept technologies that tend to set them apart from the rest of society as being different or unable to function independently. PRS with additional applications allowing for daily utilitarian use will help remove barriers to usage.

Advertising needs to show healthy active elderly as well as non-elderly utilizing PRS. This will assist in sending the message that a Personal Response System is not only for the frail elderly but has broad applications across the population spectrum. Media advertising will also increase awareness which is key to increased usage.

Cost as a perceived barrier to usage will be reduced if the industry can increase product acceptability as described above. However, there is a need to address those individuals who cannot afford the system due to lack of funds. As the industry grows the cost of the service should decline but third party coverage is vital for those elderly living near or at the poverty level. Studies show that as age increases the percent of poor and near poor living alone also increase. These elderly have one or more chronic health conditions that place them at medical risk. This same population utilizes hospital-based services at a greater rate than the non-elderly population. Research in the PRS industry continues to demonstrate compelling evidence that PRS usage is a cost effective alternative to institutional placement and that PRS can reduce hospital costs.

The industry will also have to continue to keep their hospital-based PRS programs financially healthy. Centralized monitoring operations will expand in the 90s and will offer integrated services to the health care industry beyond just Personal Response Systems. Additional product enhancements such as Lifeline's Access Package for the physically challenged will continue to expand the hospitals' market segments and thereby their financial viability.

Personal Response Systems in the U. S. will have to respond to an increasing population that does not speak English. Monitoring services must be bilingual in order to truly be available to all populations who need it.

Lastly, an added challenge for the Personal Response industry in the 90s will be to police itself in terms of quality of product and service. In an industry where medical emergencies are common and lives are at stake the quality of product and service is paramount. A user must be assured that the equipment is going to function properly every time and that service is available from a reputable company. Underwriters Laboratory certification as well as FDA certification will play an important part in assuring quality products and services in the PRS industry. As the industry grows it is vital that quality of product and service remain at the forefront. The ability for this industry to police itself in terms of quality will play a significant role in overcoming barriers to usage. We in the PRS industry in the United States need to create an industry-wide Code of Ethics which speaks to the following points:

1. The highest quality product possible.
2. Quality service to the customer.
3. Truth in advertising.
4. A goal to make the service available to all who need it.

In summation, although Personal Response Systems are relatively new in the marketplace they have made tremendous inroads over the past fifteen years. The next decade presents some difficult problems for this country in terms of its aging population and the delivery of quality, cost effective health care to all who need it. In light of these problems, the PRS industry can offer viable solutions–solutions for the U.S. health care system in helping to control and reduce the cost of health care delivery; solutions for industry in attempting to meet their employee health care needs; solutions for families who are coping with the strains of eldercare; and most important, solutions for many people who, regardless of age, could not live independently with a Personal Response System.

# REFERENCES

AARP (1987), "A Profile of Older Americans," AARP, Washington, D.C.

Bowe, Frank (1988), "Why Seniors Don't Use Technology," *Technology Review*, August/September, P.34.

Cain, Betty Ann (1987), "Effects of a Lifeline Program on Hospitalization," Presented in Partial Fulfillment of a Masters Degree in Social Work, California State University, Long Beach, California.

Dibner, Andrew S. (1982), "A National Survey of Lifeline Programs," Lifeline Systems, Inc., Watertown, Massachusetts.

Dibner, Andrew S. (1990), "Costs and Savings of Personal Emergency Response Services," Lifeline Systems, Inc., Watertown, Massachusetts.

Dibner, Andrew S. (1985), "Effects of Personal Emergency Response Services on Hospital Use," Lifeline Systems, Inc., Watertown, Massachusetts.

"Emergency Response System Demonstration Project–Preliminary Report" (1988), Coordinated Care Management Corporation, 560 Delaware Avenue, Buffalo, New York.

"Evaluation of Electronic Call Device Pilot Project" (1988), The City of New York, Human Resources Administration Medical Assistance Program, Lorie Dixon, Director, Office of Program Design.

Freedman, Jay (1989), "Abstract–Assessment of a Lifeline Program–Preliminary Findings," V.A. Medical Center, Indianapolis, Indiana.

Koch, John (1984), "Emergency Response System Assists in Discharge Planning," *Dimensions in Health Service*, Vol. 61, No. 11, Nov. 1984, P. 30-31.

"Lifeline Central Survey" (1988), Lifeline Systems, Inc., Watertown, Massachusetts.

Moschis, George P. (1989), "Older Consumer Orientations Toward Marketing Practices and Responses to New Products, A Summary Report."

Opinion Research Corporation, Washington, D.C. (1989), "Working Caregivers Report." Conducted by American Association of Retired People, Washington, D.C. and The Traveler's Foundation, Hartford, Connecticut.

Patel, Jean (1990), "Buying Behavior of the Mature Market," Lifeline Systems, Inc., Watertown, Massachusetts.

Patel, Jean (1989), "Lifeline Program Managers Survey," Lifeline Systems, Inc., Watertown, Massachusetts.

Patel, Jean (1989), "Lifeline Users Survey," Lifeline Systems, Inc., Watertown, Massachusetts.

Ruchlin, Hirsch S. and John N. Morris (1981), "Cost-Benefit Analysis of an Emergency Alarm and Response System: A Case Study of a Long-Term Care Program," *Health Services Research* 16:1 65-80.

Sherwood, Sylvia and John N. Morris (1980), "A Study of the Effects of an Emergency Alarm and Response System for the Aged: A Final Report," Grant No. HS01788, National Center for Health Services Research.

Stafford, Juliene S. and Dibner, Andrew S. (1984), "Lifeline Programs in 1984–Growth and Stability," Lifeline Systems, Inc., Watertown, Massachusetts.

# Public Financing
# for Personal Response Systems:
# A Federal Viewpoint

William F. Benson

The major publicly funded health care programs in the United States do not, for the most part, pay for emergency response systems. And, unfortunately, we don't, at the present time, have the most hospitable climate for ensuring that ERS is available to those who would benefit from them.

- Medicare, the principal source of social health insurance for the nation's elderly, does not cover ERS.
- Medicaid, the public welfare health program for the nation's poor, covers ERS, in some of the 50+ states and territories, under certain circumstance only. And, where Medicaid does cover ERS, the criteria are often so rigid it raises questions as to whether those who can get coverage are the ones who would most benefit from it.
- Other, less significant health-related services, may cover ERS on a largely *ad hoc* basis; for example through the Older Americans Act.
- Private insurance to supplement Medicare–Medigap–does not normally cover ERS. Other private health coverage, including insurance provided to retirees by their former employers, typically does not cover it.
- Of course, for those who can afford it out-of-pocket, ERS systems are readily available, if they are aware of it.

It is important to note that despite the lack of public and private insurance coverage, the growth in the use of ERS in this country is quite impressive; some 2,700 hospitals participate in ERS systems.

The lack of coverage notwithstanding, it seems that there is widespread

William F. Benson is affiliated with the Senate Labor and Human Resources Committee of the United States.

acknowledgement that this low-cost technology is of great value to those who have it:

- It is very cost-effective;
- It saves lives; and
- It supports a fundamental value of Americans, like that of citizens in the various countries represented here, to remain at home independently for as long as possible–in short, it enables people to avoid institutionalization, at least for a longer period, if not entirely.

There are other strong public policy reasons to provide ERS services, including:

- We have a shortage of nursing home beds in many parts of the country–a shortage that is likely to get worse–it seems important to ensure that beds are available for those most in need of them;
- Institutional care is very expensive–the annual cost of a nursing home stay is now over $30,000, or $82 per day *the states are already spending 50 percent of their Medicaid health care dollar on nursing home care*–it is essential that states and the federal government find every way possible to provide alternatives and minimize public expenditures on nursing homes to the greatest extent practicable; and
- The sheer demographics of the so-called "graying of America" is part of the "graying of nations."

I don't need to provide you with a litany of statistics about this phenomenon, but it is important to mention that the numbers of those aged 85 and over will simply explode over the next 25 years.

So, given these arguments as to why ERS is an important service, why isn't it covered in our principal public health care programs? I would like to offer a few thoughts about that and then give you my prognosis.

For most, the U.S. health care system is complex, confusing, costly, and fragmented, if not chaotic. In fact, many argue that it is not a system but rather a hodge-podge collection of different programs with different services, requirements, eligibility criteria, and delivery mechanisms; and so on.

*Let's start with Medicare*, our national and most comprehensive health care program for the elderly. Advocates of ERS believe that Medicare should cover this service. From a cost-savings point of view, a strong argument can be made that, in light of the extraordinary cost of hospital and emergency care, the use of ERS could prevent more serious harm and reduce medical costs in particular circumstances. Medicare, however, is essentially an acute care driven system–it has not played much of a role on the prevention side.

In 1988, Congress enacted the Medicare Catastrophic Coverage ACT (MCCA), which was hailed as the most sweeping improvements in Medicare since it was established in 1965. The new law included coverage for a prevention program–breast cancer screening. Unfortunately, the new law became the Medicare Debacle Act and, a little more than a year later, the entire Act was repealed (except for Medicaid provisions).

Unfortunately, a broader view of cost-savings potential didn't help to save key benefits. Among the various benefits repealed was a significant improvement in Medicare's nursing home (SNF) benefit which eliminated the requirement that beneficiaries had to be hospitalized for 3 days before getting the nursing home coverage. Despite anecdotal indications and the intuitive sense that forcing people into a hospital for 3 days increases costs significantly, the hard data that Medicare would save money without the 3-day requirement simply was–and is–not available. Thus, this progressive change in the law went down with the rest of the MCCA.

Many feel, and I am one of them, that attempts at reinstating these changes and other program improvements in Medicare, will have a very difficult time in the Congress and with the executive branch of government. This, coupled with the acute care bias of Medicare, makes the likelihood of adding a service such as ERS slim, in the absence of a dramatic overhaul of Medicare–which is also unlikely in the near future.

On a positive Medicare note, however, the government has been experimenting with social HMOS (S/HMO). All four of the test sites include provision of ERS.

*Next, let's look at Medicaid.* Medicaid is our program for providing health care coverage for the poor. It is a joint federal and state program, with the federal government picking up at least 50% of a state's Medicaid expenditures. In reality, Medicaid differs from state to state–Medicaid is an umbrella for 50+ different programs in the states, D.C., and the territories. And, the umbrella is full of holes.

You may have seen the front page story about Medicaid: *"Health Officials Fear Medicaid Drifting Toward Collapse."* During the past decade, the states have been forced to pick up the tab for more and more Medicaid costs. Medicaid continues to increase as a significant portion of a state's budget, paid directly by the general fund. As in the movie *Network,* the states' governors said last year "We've had enough and we're not going to take anymore," and collectively beseeched Congress and the White House to not impose any more Medicaid mandates on them.

We already have a rough road ahead in being sure that all states proceed with the programs currently required by law. For example, Congress enacted in 1987 sweeping reforms in the laws governing quality of care in nursing homes. These reforms, which place a sizeable responsibility on the states, took full effect October, 1 of 1990. There are, unfortunately, signs that implementation of this critical new law will be uneven among the states, mostly due to concerns about cost.

*The bottom line: this is a very difficult time to implement new services and requirements in the Medicaid program.* However, all is not bleak here with regard to ERS, and I will return to this momentarily.

It is essential to note that at least those who are on Medicare and Medicaid have health coverage, despite the program's limitations. In the U.S., *we have an estimated 31-37 million Americans without any health care insurance whatsoever.* Millions more are either underinsured or their coverage is vulnerable to their work or their employer's circumstances. *Medicaid covers 40% of the poor and 60% of the working poor* (Urban Institute, 1990). In sum, our health care financing and delivery system is in need of major serious work.

In a sense, however, this provides several possible scenarios for coverage of ERS and other smaller, low-cost (in the scheme of things) services, such as mammography screening.

- Include ERS as part of a major overhaul of health care coverage.
- Include ERS as part of incremental improvements–which may be an attractive/realistic alternative to overhaul.
- Opportunity to take a broad view of cost savings services such as prevention and detection services.

While I have portrayed what seems to be a fairly bleak picture, the news is not all grim. In fact, at least looking down the road, I believe there is reason to be optimistic, both on an incremental and large-scale basis.

Our budgetary woes are very serious to be sure, but so are our health care woes. We need a long-term care system. ERS is a long-term care service and should be part of any comprehensive LTC effort. Many believe we are more likely to get a LTC program in place before we effectively address the needs of 37 million uninsured Americans. Certainly, major opinion polls suggest strong support for a public LTC system.

The congressionally established *Pepper Commission*, consisting of top congressional health care leaders issued its recommendations in March, 1990 for a national LTC system, including a social insurance program for home based care. When the Pepper Commission releases its final report, I am hopeful that it will provide an important boost for ERS. Following this report, there is expected to be a flurry of legislative proposals introduced, including one by Senator Pryor. These bills will provide a key opportunity to ensure that thinking regarding LTC especially, and home and community-based care, includes ERS.

While these Bills were not likely to be enacted in 1990, they will form the basis for legislative action in the next Congress. More immediate, however, is the strong possibility of enactment this year of S. 1942, Senators Rockefeller, Pryor and others' bill to allow states the option of choosing to provide home and community-based care, rather than go through the bureaucratic and difficult special waiver program (Section 2176). The Bill–the Medicaid Home and Community Care Options Act–would enable the DHHS secretary to include ERS as a service a state *could* opt to provide.

We have been working closely with Dr. Dibner on an amendment to the Rockefeller Bill to explicitly cite ERS as a service that *can* be provided though not mandated. Congressman Rinaldo in the house has offered similar legislation. The single significant key to enactment of S. 1942 (with our amendment of course) is the outcome of the budget summit currently underway between Congress and the Administration. That will, of course, effect a whole lot more than S. 1942.

It is important to note, and Dr. Dibner can rattle off the figures with ease, a number of states already provide ERS under their sec. 2176 waiver programs–albeit typically on a limited basis. The states' right to seek a sec. 2176 waiver and cover ERS, or do so under their Medicaid personal care option, if approved by the secretary, if they exercise it, would remain intact with S. 1942.

*ERS may have a much stronger possibility as the development of home and community-based care moves forward.*

There is another parallel major legislative track underway in Congress: overhaul of our nation's housing policy.

- 80% reduction of HUD housing during Reagan years.
- *S. 566* (Cranston) and house legislation: *A major component is a strong supportive services component* to address the needs of those "aging in place" and the disabled.
- We have a great deal to learn from other countries. In reading the abstracts for this symposium, we saw the emphasis in some places of linking ERS with housing services.
- We're working on *amendments to the housing reform legislation. This presents a strong opportunity for including ERS coverage.*
- Downside: Adding to Housing programs would perpetuate our already disjointed health and LTC delivery system. But, could provide a source of coverage for some persons.

The 1991 Reauthorization of OAA provides an opportunity to expand availability of ERS.

Before closing, I would like to mention briefly several key challenges facing those of you advocating for greater coverage and utilization of ERS in the U.S.

- *Cost Issues.* We need hard data to show cost effectiveness and overall efficacy of ERS. There must be much more than we have now–a broad potential for real savings.
- *"Woodwork Effect."* If there was more government coverage, would this lead to an over-use of the service?
- *The DME "Taint"*–There is congressional concern about unethical marketing practices, particularly if ERS is distributed as "durable medical equipment."

In sum, advocates for ERS have not made an overwhelmingly compelling case for ERS, on cost or human terms–why is it necessary that government explicitly cover ERS? Moreover, it is essential that advocates mobilize in the states and build allies, particularly in the LTC community.

# ERS as a Community Outreach Service from a Nursing Home

Betty J. Schantz

## INTRODUCTION AND OVERVIEW

The United Presbyterian Home (UPH), located at Woodbury, New York (approximately 30 miles east of New York City on Long Island) is a dedicated non-sectarian home which provides comprehensive health care and skilled nursing facilities in a tranquil wooded setting. In 1983 UPH realized that additional assistance for the elderly and frail was needed beyond the limited capacity of the home itself. Lifeline Systems was approached to determine if its emergency response services (ERS) could be an answer to UPH's planned outreach support program. The result was a strong affirmative. In an aging society, with rapidly increasing medical and housing costs, a Lifeline to elderly and frail persons at a modest cost was considered a godsend.

UPH's Lifeline program has been growing ever since its inception in 1983, now numbering over 1,300 active subscribers. The limitations on its continued rapid growth are the starting costs associated with additional new units and the expanded demand for staff to provide the needed additional marketing, installation, service and administration capacity. A benefit from the Lifeline Program to the UPH is the awareness created among the subscribers of the existence and expertise of the Home as a reliable provider of full time health care, should the need ever arise.

## DEMOGRAPHIC INFORMATION

In 1980, the National census revealed that over 2,600,000 persons lived in the Nassau/Suffolk County area of which more than 214,000 were over

Betty J. Schantz is affiliated the United Presbyterian Home, United States.

60 years of age. In this year's census it is almost certain that the total population will have increased and the percentag. of the elderly to the total population will have increased even more. It has been estimated that the number of the elderly will rise by at least one third. This expanding trend of the population and the elderly foreshadows a growing problem on Long Island.

Currently at UPH 95% of our subscribers are over 60 years of age. Eighty two percent (82%) are female and 3% are considered handicapped, referring to those who are under 60 years of age who have either muscular dystrophy or are paraplegics.

## TECHNOLOGY AND SERVICE

The communicator equipment used by UPH is the RC400. Lifetrac software (management information system, compatible with the IBM-PC-AT), AccPac (accounts receivable software), and a Wang word processor are also used. Phone calls are monitored on a 24 hour per day basis every day of the year by a dedicated and trained team of UPH employees located at Flushing House, which is an adult home for independent living in Queens County and operated by UPH. Since that facility already provided 24 hour security services for its 320 residents, and had a well-trained staff conditioned to dealing with the emergency needs of the frail and elderly on a face to face basis, it made it both advantageous and cost effective to have the Lifeline Response Center located in the Flushing House Security Office.

When a Lifeline subscriber is in need of help a personal help button, that is worn on their person, is pushed which sends a signal through a toll-tree telephone number to the response center in a matter of seconds which then sets off an alarm and records it on the RC400 tape (see Photo). The subscriber information is automatically viewed on the PC screen. The Lifeline staff member pushes a button on the computer which enables automatic voice contact with the subscriber. If this call is not answered by the subscriber another call to a designated responder is made, asking that person to physically verify the nature of the original alarm call. If the designated responder is unable to be reached or if they are not able to make contact with the subscriber a call to the police (on the emergency 911 line) is made. This procedure assures that help will be on location with minimum delay.

PHOTO. Subscriber holding Lifeline portable help button.

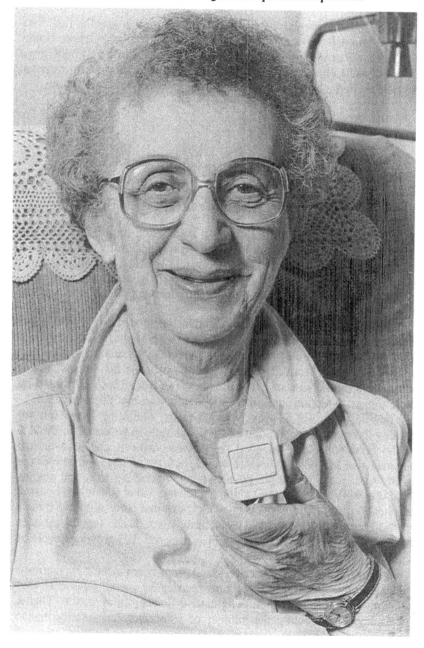

## *ECONOMICS*

The Lifeline Emergency Response Service program was the first community outreach service sponsored by the United Presbyterian Home. Seed money was initially provided by the UPH along with a $15,000 grant from Nassau County. The acceptance of external funding led to certain restrictions in the Nassau County fee structure which is shown below.

| *Income per Yr.* *In Dollars* | *Monthly Fee* *In Dollars* |
|---|---|
| Under 4,000 | 10 |
| 4,000-7,000 | 15 |
| 7,001-10,000 | 20 |
| Over 10,000 | 25 |

A refundable deposit of $25 and an installation fee of $50 was also established. Private subscriber fees for a Non-Voice unit have been set at $32.50 per month with a $32.50 refundable security deposit and for a Voice unit $40.00 respectively with $75.00 installation fee for both types of units. Reduced rate fees represent approximately 15% of our total fee structure.

Sometimes public support is available, such as Long Term Home Health Care (Lombardi Program) associated with Medicaid, or the regular Medicaid program if they fall within the coverage guidelines.

Billing is done from the United Lifeline office. Bills are sent out to subscribers on the first of every month. "Test your Unit" is printed on each invoice to remind subscribers of the importance of this procedure.

The 1980 National Census provided many interesting local facts regarding the economic condition of the population. In Nassau County 44% of the households that included persons 65 years of age or over had incomes over $15,000 per year. However, in 6.1% of these households the family was living below the poverty level. According to recent studies there is a five year or greater waiting list to enter either subsidized housing or a health care facility. This clearly indicates that more support services for the aged will be required in the coming years. These support services must be made available but they will require parallel growing levels of funding.

Funding comes from subscribers and from benevolent contributions. Greater number of subscribers not only reduces the overall support service problem but additionally, permits greater efficiency in operation. This is not to say that doubling the number of subscribers necessarily means doubling the required number of staff members, however, UPH does from time to time, review staffing to ensure that efficiency is monitored as the program grows. Receiving outright gifts from charitable organizations is another means of helping the ERS program grow. Both avenues of revenue are being pursued.

The major sources for grants and gifts have come from Nassau County, private corporations, service organizations, churches and individuals. The most generous of these have been Nassau County and the Grumman Corporation. Contributions are received only by expending considerable effort to get them. The results were achieved through the use of official letters, personal contacts and presentations. Soliciting is a never-ending endeavor and is usually fruitful only in proportion to the real effort made.

Getting the "Lifeline" message out to the public, to generate interest for new subscribers, is another task that must be undertaken with spirit. Some of the methods we have used at UPH include:

- *Newspapers*–Pictures and words similar to our brochure.
- *Local Radio/TV*–Personal appearances in a talk show setting.
- *Churches/Temples*–Letter (with brochure and return address reply card) requesting opportunity to meet with leaders to explain project, followed up by a slide presentation. A request is also usually made that insert material be included in any bulletin or newsletter.
- *Service Clubs* (Rotary, Lions, Kiwanis, etc.) A letter is forwarded requesting the opportunity to make a slide presentation and that consideration be given towards the purchase of a Lifeline unit.
- *Doctors*–Letter requesting the opportunity to visit and explain the program and permission to leave an explanatory brochure for patients.
- *Senior Centers*–Letter requesting the opportunity to make a slide presentation to be followed by a question and answer period.
- *Hospitals*–Appointments were made with hospitals, within a 150 mile radius, to meet with administrative and social service departments to explain the program and UPH's service commitment. Brochures were left and many referrals were made directly to UPH. Some hospitals prefer to make use of UPH's services while they publicize that they offer Lifeline. They then do their own billing.
- *Advertisements*–Yellow Pages, Long Island Business Fairs, Health Fairs, Handicapped Newspapers.

Experience has shown that in attracting and obtaining new subscribers the most effective methods were the presentations and personal recommendations.

## OPERATIONS

United Lifeline answers approximately 1000 calls per month. While only 10% of these are actual emergencies, practically all are due to falls and not being able to get up by themselves, and 12% are related to user inactivity primarily because of forgetfulness or the inability to reset due to death. The remaining 78% are false alarms which we use to our advantage by treating them as a substitute for our regular monthly test calls. There have been nearly 2700 installations made to date with just over 1300 currently active subscribers. The roughly 50% turnover rate in seven years is an interesting statistic. The average length of service per subscriber is about twelve months. Incoming inquiries currently average 150 per month, with the major sources of subscriber contact coming from:

- Subscriber referral
- Doctors
- Senior Centers
- Hospitals
- Radio/Television
- Visiting Nurses
- Social Workers

When the subscriber level passed the 300 level, it was found necessary to add additional staff to monitor the around the clock activity, plus all the other tasks. These included making monthly test calls, updating subscriber information and verifying that their equipment was operating properly.

The purchase of "Lifetrac" software made subscriber monitoring much more efficient in all phases of the operation. This software permitted a great improvement in gathering statistical data, such as:

- subscriber primary diagnosis
- age
- sex
- referral source
- types of emergencies

This information is necessary for our monthly reports. Our inventory and record keeping was further enhanced by additional software developed at the United Presbyterian Home. This software now allows us to keep exact track of all our units and their history plus the battery change schedules.

## *INSTALLATION PROCEDURE OF A LIFELINE UNIT*

After a telephone call comes in inquiring about United Lifeline we ask "How did you hear about us." We then say, "do you want me to explain the service or send you a brochure." After we have established that they want the information we ask their name and the name of the person for whom they want the service, address and telephone number, how they heard about us and how many telephone instruments they have (required information for installer) and arrange an appointment for one of our staff to go to their home. When the home visit is made we go through a detailed explanation on how the unit works and assure the subscriber that it is not difficult and make them feel comfortable with its operation. We advise them that since the personal help button is waterproof they can even wear it when bathing. This is certainly a plus since we found from statistics that most accidents happen in the bathroom. We proceed to ask medical history, and any pertinent information on their responders. This data is then called into the office to be installed into Lifetrac so that the subscriber is immediately on line. While this is being done the telephone installer is doing the required telephone work. When his work is completed we do an actual demonstration with the response center at which time they "welcome" the subscriber to United Lifeline. Upon returning to the office we create a file and input into our computer inventory. A thank you letter with an explanation of the procedure is sent to the responders and doctor.

## *OTHER STAFF ACTIVITIES*

Other activities are carried out by the office staff, consisting of two full time employees and three part-time employees. The more important of these are as follows:

- Monthly report for administration
- Battery updates
- Pickups
- Malfunction changes
- Clean units
- Billing–Account Receivables and Payable
- Insert bills and envelopes for mailings
- Inquiry letters
- Soliciting for presentations and funding

- Prepare promotional articles for Home paper
- Organize and host annual Lifeline Tea

Additionally, we have occasional volunteers help with light office work and telephone inquiries.

## SOCIAL TEA

As an example of outreach, once a year, usually in September, UPH sponsors a United Lifeline Tea to invite subscribers and their responders to the resident facility to enjoy hors d'oeuvre, sandwiches, cake, coffee, etc. This gives them a chance to meet the Lifeline staff and other subscribers who have the one thing in common, Lifeline. It also offers an opportunity for them to inspect the UPH facility as a possible future residence.

This social event has been run for several years now with great success. Naturally, only a small percentage actually attend due to varied circumstances. There is a certain comraderie between the "old folks" and with some outside entertainment as well as their own in singing, story telling, dancing, etc., and a wonderful time is had by all. Gifts and recognition are given to the subscriber that has been on the system the longest and the same to the eldest. They have come to look forward to this event each year.

## BENEFITS OF ERS

The benefits of Emergency Response Services have been found to be spread over a wide spectrum of human concern. These benefits include psychological, medical, social and cost, each of which has a significant impact on the subscriber and his/her family. More specifically the United Lifeline program:

- Helps elders maintain their independence in their own homes and neighborhoods with increased security, confidence and dignity.
- Reduces the sense of isolation for the elderly by providing a feeling of security. They know they can get help quickly in case of need.
- Prevents premature institutionalization of frail persons by assuring them and those concerned with their welfare that a wide range of medical and social services are available to them at the push of a button.

- Assures that older adults have easy access to emergency services in case of an accident or illness, giving family members greater peace of mind.
- Connects those who are socially isolated with protective services in case of crime or other environmental stress.
- Establishes links and coordinates with existing services so that United Lifeline becomes part of a comprehensive plan of service.
- Reduces the cost of support of elderly people by providing the level of service needed at a moderate cost, where care at a total health care facility is neither required or desired.

## EXPECTED FUTURE DEVELOPMENTS

Currently we own 1700 units with 1300 in the field and an additional 150 is expected by the end of this year. It is anticipated that the UPH will continue to increase at this rate in the foreseeable future. In the very near future, the home is also planning on building a senior citizen cluster housing development to be known as "Stonewall Farms." The ninety eight individual apartments will be built on 9.8 acres professionally landscaped with trees and shrubbery. United Lifeline will be available to tenants at an additional charge to provide assistance in their apartments and common area in the event of a health emergency.

## FUTURE TECHNICAL DEVELOPMENT

Our current technical environment is centered around the Lifetrac software, RC400 operating in an IBM PC286.

While this equipment served its purpose to get started in this program UPH is now looking to upgrade our system to handle potential growth in all facets of this operation.

This could be done by upgrading to a PC386 DOS machine which would improve both storage capacity and speed at a reasonable additional cost.

Our system could then be converted into a multi-work station arrangement or what is called Local Area Networking (LAN). This would, for example, allow us to make monthly test calls without interfering with emergency response calls, as well as other administrative functions all from the same information data base.

It is our belief that such a system would enhance our total operation while maintaining our integrity in meeting the challenge of future growth and performance.

## CONCLUSION

What was true many years ago about what United Presbyterian Home stands for--providing that extra measure of care and concern to its residents--is still true today, but in today's world one has to look outside the Home as well to keep up with the growing elderly population and its needs.

It is for this reason we at UPH are striving to meet this demand by looking seriously into all facets of health care and outreach programs.

Lifeline happens to be one of the greatest potential sources to answer this need in the 90's and while we still adhere to the simple truths that "a house may give shelter but a home provides warmth" we are dedicated through Lifeline to extending that "warm feeling" into private homes as well.

# SUMMARY AND DISCUSSION

# Personal Response Services
# Present and Future

Andrew S. Dibner

## PRESENT STATUS OF PRS

Approximately fifteen years ago a new service appeared on the health care scene, applying modern communication technology to the need for protection for elderly and disabled persons living alone. Personal response systems (PRS) send an automatic phone call for help if a person at home cannot use normal means for signalling an emergency.

PRS technology began to be applied in many countries, but there was no forum for international exchange of information. The American Lifeline Institute recognized this need and invited leaders in the PRS field from 12 countries to present papers and exchange information. Eighteen speakers provided rich information about the state of the art of PRS, its demand, economics, and methods of operation. Representatives from government, academia, health services, social services, and business from England, West Germany, Canada, Holland, Sweden, Denmark, Scotland, Wales, Japan, New Zealand, Israel and the United States presented to a fascinated audience.

Andrew S. Dibner is affiliated with American Lifetime Institute, Newton, MA 02159.

Clearly the growth and acceptance of PRS internationally is being fueled by ubiquitous population changes. Through better nutrition and health care the oldest old are living longer. More of them need help in maintaining independent living. Across nations, there is consensus that promoting independent living for the elderly through home and community care is preferable to institutional care. Whether and under what circumstances home care is economically advantageous is still an unanswered question, but the Symposium presenters agreed that home care is the more humane solution.

Enter PRS. Here there is clear agreement. Presenters agreed that the sense of security given to users and their families by this means of immediate contact with help can be a potent force in helping people remain living alone despite frailties or potentially dangerous medical conditions.

The technology for PRS seems to be quite similar across countries. Home equipment includes an automatic telephone dialer/reporter with 2-way voice capability, activated either by a permanently mounted button or a portable radio transmitter worn on the person. The dialer communicates with either a local or regional emergency response center operating 24 hours a day.

Some systems have employed an additional "passive" type of alarm responsive to a person's unusual inactivity. Speakers disagreed as to the value of passive alarms, mainly because they are often seen by users as an intrusion on their privacy, e.g., if it is keyed to use of the toilet or refrigerator. It is also reason for a high rate of false alarms. However, some felt false alarms, in general, have some benefits. They provide practice for the user and are considered to be a positive way for the user to remain actively aware of the system's purpose and function.

All presenters prefer wireless portable help buttons which are waterproof, light and aesthetically designed, two-way voice communication, use of regional response centers, and the integration of PRS with other medical and social services.

Costs of PRS varied less than one would expect. Prices ranged from $600-$1200 for home equipment, and monthly monitoring fees ranged between $10-$40. In countries with national medical plans PRS is subsidized heavily, but, increasingly, subsidies are declining and private pay increasing.

The United States is unique in its use of hospitals to distribute PRS, as it is in its funding which, to date, has been largely private rather than government sponsored. A new trend in the United States suggests that there will be increasing inclusion of PRS in Medicaid home and community care services and in supportive services for public housing of the frail elderly.

Where public sources pay for PRS screening referral of PRS users is most often based on medical criteria and functional capacity, not on age. History of falling or having cardiac or mobility problems were the most common criteria used for referral.

Across all countries the primary users of PRS are women in their 70's and 80's living alone, burdened usually with cardiac and musculoskeletal problems and subject to falls. The gender difference in the use of PRS reflects different longevity rates for men and women.

Across nations the most significant obstacle to acceptance of PRS by users is denial of need. Older people most often do not feel themselves particularly in need of help, as they consider themselves neither more disabled nor less competent than others. Economic constraints are, of course, another obstacle to PRS use, but become less of an obstacle when PRS is fully or partially subsidized.

One marketing issue posed as a problem at the Symposium was the association of PRS with the burglar alarm industry, which, because of unethical techniques involving eliciting fear in their advertising, has given it a bad reputation. Similarly, if PRS is associated with the "old" it immediately runs the risk of bearing all the negative stereotypes of aging, popularly called "agism." Older persons do not wish to be considered old, nor do younger persons want that pejorative label even though they may be in need of PRS protection. Thus, linking PRS to the aged makes for marketing problems.

Monitoring PRS signals is another complex topic across nations. Whether monitoring should be local, regional or national is a matter for debate. Some argue for local response centers which have greater understanding of local circumstances, so that information can be expeditiously used in counseling and referring users. Others counter by defending larger monitoring centers, claiming their greater efficiency through greater volume and better trained and supervised, professional staff.

It is fairly well agreed that family, neighbors and volunteers can adequately serve as the first line of responders in an emergency if backed up by professional medical help if needed, rather than using ambulances or other emergency teams as the first line of response. Informal responders are trusted and research has shown that they can resolve emergencies themselves in more than 60% of cases, thus providing an economical resource. It is important, too, to keep as much of a human element in the system as possible. It was reported by several presenters that the frequency of family and friend's visits and care did not diminish with a person using PRS, despite the fears of some critics.

The growth of PRS has been fueled from its start by an interesting combination of private and public forces, with for-profit, technology-driven companies promoting a product which is genuinely desired, and by public not-for-profit agencies, most of which are not accustomed to purchasing electronic devices. Although early PRS development in some of the nations represented here was characterized by inefficient public planning and purchasing, as the field matures public purchasers have become more sophisticated and are demanding reliable equipment, competitive prices, uniform standards and consumer guides. Standards which will establish minimal functions and possibly compatibility of operating modes are being developed by SENELEC and independently in the U.K. In the U.S.A. the Underwriters Laboratory has developed safety and reliability standards for "Home Care Signalling Equipment."

Experts from all countries agree that PRS is cost effective in saving institutional health care costs, although the only hard research on cost savings has been done in the United States, as described in the chapter by Christina Montgomery. Others have pursued research on use of the system and client satisfaction, with uniformly positive results. Each country expects that PRS will not only continue to grow to serve the security needs of frail elderly, but may in addition be used for medical monitoring and for other security tasks and populations as well.

## PRS IN THE FUTURE

The future of PRS will continue to be driven by the two forces which shaped its growth to this point: pressure to help an increasingly growing older population to live securely and comfortably at home, and continued progress in electronic and telephone technology. Auto-dialing, memory-phones, and telephone answering machines are commonplace today though only a dream two decades ago. What's next? Probably a very smart in-home combination of telephone and computer terminal which will have speech recognition and generation, video and audio output, data storage, automatic communication capability, and the capability to control many aspects of life at home. When that kind of communication and control technology in the home gets linked to miniaturized sensors, transmitters, and receivers which can be carried with a person anywhere, the ideal will be real–no one need be out of touch, no matter where they are.

PRS in the future will include more services than making emergency calls. Even now PRS is monitoring for smoke, extremes in temperature, and gas or water dangers. Medical monitoring and transmission of medical data is available, though as yet little used, as is monitoring and control of in-home health care equipment and environmental controls. Also the use of PRS for reducing a sense of isolation and producing social reassurance is here but not yet fully realized.

PRS has the capability of providing a permanent communication link from home to an administrative center which is not only a monitoring station but also an intelligent information bank. It has what it takes to be the key to integrative management of home care services. PRS staff and equipment could monitor and manage the flow of information about patient status, prescribed services, scheduling of services and provision of those services. For disabled, frail or ill persons at home who need many services, medications and equipment, efficient information and management control is essential.

In the future, the marketing and distribution of PRS will be changing. Each country will work within its cultural values and within its political and economic system to provide greater market penetration of the frail and not-so-frail elderly groups; but there is need for PRS by many other groups including unsupervised children, younger disabled persons, and anyone perceived as vulnerable in a threatening environment, such as employees alone at night or those subject to marital violence or racial harassment. Until these problems are solved in more widespread social improvements, this technology can protect society's weakest, most vulnerable members. Equipment must be developed to meet the special needs of these groups, and marketing and distribution needs to sensitively present PRS to assure its acceptance as a new aid.

Across the nations, the funding of PRS will continue to be shared by public and private sources. As third party payors (insurance companies, employers, and government organizations) realize the cost savings generated by PRS, they will increase their coverage of the service. At the same time private markets will continue to expand as manufacturers and distributors reach out to present them with attractive equipment and service to meet their needs.

International exchange of information such as that which was stimulated by the American Lifeline Institute's *First International Symposium on Emergency Response Services for Frail Persons Living Alone* will lead to further conferences and, hopefully, to a formal international planning group to include both manufacturers and consumers. This book is one step in the process of promoting this international dialogue.

# Index

Tabular material indicated by a "t" following a page number; figures indicated by "fig."

AARP, Profile of Older Americans
217
Access to person's home 185-186
Actionline, in the Netherlands 102
Activities of Daily Living (ADL)24
Advertising
need for 220
by UPH 233
Age statistics in Denmark 36-37
Aged households, increase of
82,84,85t
Alarm coverage in England 181-186
Alarm-call systems 130-133
Alarms in the UK
advertising 178
dispersed 179
history of, 178-179
Alarm system
in Israel 70-72
in New Zealand 129
Alarm system research in England
180,195,197-198
American Lifeline Institute
2-3,239,243
Attitudes toward ERS 7-8,9,78

Barriers to usage
denial of need, 215-218
lack of awareness, 217-218
Benefits
for caregiver 210-211
financial 211-212
for health care system 212-215

in Israel 78-80
psychological 97,120,145-146
in UPH program 236-237
British Standards Institution 168
Building Automation
by Canadian Automated Building
Association 19

Call system in Denmark 39
Care and intercare phone systems
137-138,140-143,146-147
Care provision
'Caring for People' White Paper
165
Categories of need for ERS 75,77
Characteristics of ERS 173
Charity ethic 127
Code of ethics, needed221
Community Alarms Programme
by Help the Aged 191-193
Community alarm systems
in England 191-199
in Scotland 149,151-158
Community based non-profit
program 17-18
Community care policies 179
Community outreach service, ERS as
229,232
Community systems, need of 28
Contact persons
choice of
in Canada 28-29
in England 185
in Germany 62,65-66

Printed in the United States
by Baker & Taylor Publisher Services